MULTIPLE CHOICE QUESTIONS TUTOR

ANATOMY, PHYSIOLOGY AND PATHOLOGY FOR RADIOGRAPHERS

Michael Brown FCR, TDCR
Principal, Edinburgh School of Diagnostic Radiography

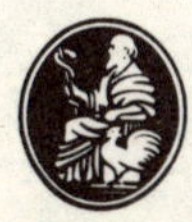

WILLIAM HEINEMANN MEDICAL BOOKS
London

William Heinemann Medical Books,
22 Bedford Square,
London WC1B 3HH

ISBN: 0–433–04510–8

First published 1987

Typeset by TecSet Ltd., Wallington, Surrey.
Printed and bound in Great Britain by Biddles Limited, Guildford.

CONTENTS

PREFACE

A 50 item multiple choice question paper was introduced into the Anatomy, Physiology and Pathology examination for Part 1 of the Diploma of the College of Radiographers in October 1982.

It is essential that the techniques used in this type of examination are familiar to both examiner and examinee: the examiner so that an objective means of assessment is provided, and the examinee so that a knowledge of the subject matter can be fairly displayed without being bothered by question format or type of question.

An objective type multiple choice examination paper is a very good instrument for testing a limited but important range of ability. If it is accepted that the aim in the examination is to test these abilities by the best possible means so that a professional profile of each examinee might be formed, the techniques of the multiple choice examination are appropriate and efficient.

This book contains 215 questions based on the two educationally accepted types used in the examination, each presented in a separate section. The specific instructions for each type are given at the beginning of the section.

For convenience each section is subdivided into related topic areas, with a representative sample of questions related to that topic. The majority of answers are accompanied by an explanation together with a reference from a standard text-book for immediate feedback and possible later revision. The list of references (*A–W*) is given at the end of the book.

This book would not have been possible without the consent of the College of Radiographers and I am indebted to them for permission to use material from the question bank.

I would like to mention the many radiographers who compiled the original questions, and then amended them; the hundreds of students who tested the items, and then helped validate the tests; the faithful few who agonised over every Facility Value, Index of Discrimination and Reliability Coefficient to produce the question bank.

Finally my appreciation to Mrs Sandra Killean for commenting on the original draft and Mrs Doreen Keith for typing the manuscript.

SECTION 1

Introduction

Each question consists of a stem, followed by 5 options.
ONE of the options is the best choice for the particular stem and is termed the KEY. The other 4 options are termed DISTRACTORS.

In this section the Key is denoted by the term TRUE, the Distractors by the term FALSE.

In the examination, candidates are required to mark their selection in ONE of 5 boxes labelled **A** to **E** inclusive.

The instruction that introduces this type of question in the examination is as follows:

Each of the following questions or incomplete statements is followed by 5 suggested answers. Select the ONE which is best in each case.

1.1 CYTOLOGY AND EMBRYOLOGY

1 An erythrocyte is a:

A. red blood cell.
B. white blood cell.
C. platelet.
D. neutrophil.
E. plasma cell.

2 With reference to localised cells, the term 'necrosis' means:

A. excessive growth.
B. inflammation.
C. degeneration.
D. death.
E. regeneration.

Answers overleaf

1A
TRUE—A red blood cell is termed an erythrocyte. Reference *A*, p. 131.

1B
FALSE—White blood cells are termed either granulocytes, lymphocytes or monocytes. Reference *A*, p. 135.

1C
FALSE—A platelet is termed a thrombocyte. Reference *A*, p. 137.

1D
FALSE—A neutrophil is one of the three groups of granulocyte. Reference *A*, p. 136.

1E
FALSE—Plasma cells are:

a) large oval cells found in soft connective tissue. Reference *A*, p. 5.

b) derived from B-type lymphocytes and produce immunoglobulins. Reference *C*, p. 75.

2A
FALSE—Excessive growth of localised cells is termed hyperplasia. The main causes are chronic irritation or hormonal imbalance. Reference *C*, p. 161.

2B
FALSE—Inflammation is the dynamic processes by which living tissues react to injury. Reference *C*, p. 27.

2C
FALSE—Degeneration is a visible change that occurs in cells as a result of a damaging process. Reference *C*, p. 3.

2D
TRUE—Necrosis is the death of cells whilst still forming part of the living body. Reference *C*, p. 3.

2E
FALSE—Regeneration is the restoration of epithelial tissue mainly as part of the healing process. Reference *C*, p. 84.

3 Schwann cells are found in the:

A. astrocytes.
B. neurilemma.
C. oligodendrocytes.
D. synapses.
E. dendrites.

4 Bacteria which are harmful to man are classed as:

A. toxins.
B. antigens.
C. commensals.
D. pathogens.
E. antibodies.

Answers overleaf

3A

FALSE—Astrocytes are one type of neuroglia the branches of which terminate on neurone cell bodies or blood capillaries. Reference *D*, p. 283.

3B

TRUE—The neurilemma is the thin membrane of the Schwann cell which envelopes the nerve cell axon along its length. Reference *D*, p. 285.

3C

FALSE—Oligodendrocytes are another type of neuroglia found mainly in the white matter of the central nervous system. Reference *D*, p. 283.

3D

FALSE—The synapses are the junctions between neurones. Reference *D*, p. 291.

3E

FALSE—Dendrites are branched processes of a neurone which receive impulses and conduct them towards the cell body. Reference *D*, p. 285.

4A

FALSE—Toxins are poisonous proteins produced by pathogenic bacteria. Reference *D*, p. 540.

4B

FALSE—Antigens are chemical substances whose introduction causes the body to produce specific antibodies. Reference *D*, p. 543.

4C

FALSE—A commensal is an organism which lives in or with another but does not cause injury to the host. Reference *B*, p. 395.

4D

TRUE—Bacteria are organisms which, when disease-producing, are called pathogens. Reference *D*, p. 540.

4E

FALSE—Antibodies are proteins produced by the body in response to the presence of an antigen. Reference *D*, p. 544.

5 Lymphatic capillaries are lined with:

A. ciliated epithelium.
B. endothelium.
C. mesothelium.
D. stratified epithelium.
E. transitional epithelium.

6 The nucleus of a mammalian cell contains:

A. chromosomes.
B. mitochondria.
C. lysosomes.
D. vacuoles.
E. centrosomes.

Answers overleaf

5A
FALSE—Ciliated epithelium is simple columnar epithelium where the cells have cilia. It can be found in the upper respiratory tract and the uterine (fallopian) tubes. Reference *D*, pp. 81 and 83.

5B
TRUE—Endothelium is similar to simple squamous epithelium and lines the heart, blood and lymph vessels, and forms the walls of capillaries. Reference *D*, pp. 81 and 83.

5C
FALSE—Mesothelium is similar to simple squamous epithelium but lines the thoracic and abdominopelvic cavities. Reference *D*, pp. 81 and 82.

5D
FALSE—Stratified epithelium consists of at least two layers and is for protection. Reference *D*, pp. 84 and 85.

5E
FALSE—Transitional epithelium is a type of stratified epithelium that allows distension, and can be found in the urinary bladder. Reference *D*, pp. 85 and 87.

6A
TRUE—Chromosomes are the shortened chromatin material found in the nucleus. Reference *D*, p. 62.

6B
FALSE—Mitochondria are small rod-shaped structures found throughout the cytoplasm. Reference *D*, p. 65.

6C
FALSE—Lysosomes are membrane-enclosed spheres found in the cytoplasm. Reference *D*, p. 66.

6D
FALSE—Vacuoles are fluid-filled cavities within the cytoplasm. Reference *D*, p. 66.

6E
FALSE—A centrosome is a dense area of cytoplasm found near the nucleus, but external to it. Reference *D*, p.66.

7 The most numerous cells in the blood are:

A. granular leucocytes.
B. erythrocytes.
C. lymphocytes.
D. thrombocytes (platelets).
E. eosinophils.

8 The function of mitochondria is to:

A. excrete the waste products of cell metabolism.
B. generate energy for the cell.
C. carry the cell characteristics on to daughter cells.
D. break down protein.
E. initiate cell division.

Answers overleaf

7A
FALSE—The total white cell count has a range of 4–11 000 cells per cubic millimetre (mm^3) ($4–11 \times 10^9/l$), the average being $8000/mm^3$ ($8 \times 10^9/1$). The granular leucocytes constitute approximately 70% of these — $5600/mm^3$ ($5.6 \times 10^9/1$). Reference *F*, pp. 16 and 17.

7B
TRUE—The erythrocyte count per cubic millimetre is approximately 5 million ($5 \times 10^{12}/l$), 4.8 in females ($4.8 \times 10^{12}/l$) 5.4 in males ($5.4 \times 10^{12}/l$); they are the most numerous cells in the blood. Reference *F*, p. 7.

7C
FALSE—Lymphocytes constitute approximately 25% of the total white cell count — $2000/mm^3$ ($2 \times 10^9/l$). Reference *F*, p. 17.

7D
FALSE—There are 250 000 platelets per cubic millimetre of blood ($250 \times 10^9/l$). Reference *F*, p. 18.

7E
FALSE—Eosinophils constitute approximately 4% of the total white cell count — $300/mm^3$ ($0.3 \times 10^9/1$). Reference *F*, p. 17

8A
FALSE—The products of cell metabolism are excreted by secretory vacuoles. Reference *D*, p. 54.

8B
TRUE—Mitochondria contain enzymes involved in energy-releasing reactions to allow cellular activity. Reference *D*, p. 65.

8C
FALSE—The hereditary information is contained as a segment of a DNA molecule that is found within the nucleus. Reference *D*, p. 62.

8D
FALSE—Protein breakdown is performed by enzymes found in lysosomes. Reference *D*, p. 66.

8E
FALSE—The centrosome is responsible for initiating cell division. Reference *D*, p. 66 and 69.

9 Transitional epithelium is found in the:

A. gall bladder.
B. pharynx.
C. urinary bladder.
D. oesophagus.
E. uterus.

10 A gamete is:

A. the embryonic stage of a gonad.
B. a fertilised ovum.
C. a cell with half the normal number of chromosomes.
D. part of the chromosome chain.
E. a stage in embryonic development.

Answers overleaf

9A
FALSE—The gall bladder is lined with simple columnar epithelium containing goblet cells. Reference *D*, p. 83.

9B
FALSE—The upper part of the pharynx (nasopharynx) is lined with pseudostratified ciliated epithelium. The remainder of the pharynx (oro- and laryngopharynx) is lined with stratified squamous epithelium. Reference *D*, p. 557.

9C
TRUE—The urinary bladder is lined with transitional epithelium to allow expansion from within. Reference *D*, p. 87.

9D
FALSE—The oesophagus is lined with stratified squamous epithelium to give protection. Reference *D*, p. 81 and 84.

9E
FALSE—The uterus is lined with simple columnar epithelium to form a mucous membrane. Reference *D*, pp. 724 and 725.

10A
FALSE—Reference *D*, p. 742.

10B
FALSE—A fertilised ovum is called a zygote. Reference *D*, p. 745.

10C
TRUE—A cell with half the normal number of chromosomes, either an ovum or a spermatozoon, is called a gamete. Reference *D*, p. 742.

10D
FALSE—The name for part of a chromosome chain is a gene. Reference *D*, p. 69.

10E
FALSE—Reference *D*, p. 742.

11 How many chromosomes are there in the nucleus of a human cell?

A. 16.
B. 26.
C. 38.
D. 46.
E. 52.

12 The ectoderm of the embryo forms:

A. muscles.
B. skin and hair.
C. the epithelial lining of the stomach.
D. blood and blood vessels.
E. skeletal tissues.

Answers overleaf

11A
FALSE—Reference *D*, p. 742.

11B
FALSE—Reference *D*, p. 742.

11C
FALSE—Reference *D*, p. 742.

11D
TRUE—The human chromosome number is 46. Reference *D*, p. 742.

11E
FALSE—Reference *D*, p. 742.

12A
FALSE—Muscles are produced from the mesoderm. Reference *D*, p. 750.

12B
TRUE—The ectoderm forms the skin and hair. Reference *D*, p. 750.

12C
FALSE—The epithelial lining of the stomach is produced by the endoderm. Reference *D*, p. 750.

12D
FALSE—The blood and blood vessels are produced from the mesoderm. Reference *D*, p. 750.

12E
FALSE—Skeletal tissue is produced from the mesoderm. Reference *D*, p. 750.

13 The average life span of red blood cells is:

A. 40 days.
B. 60 days.
C. 80 days.
D. 120 days.
E. 140 days.

14 The outermost layer of the epidermis contains:

A. tactile nerves.
B. sweat glands.
C. blood vessels.
D. keratin.
E. melanin.

Answers overleaf

13A
FALSE—Reference *E*, p. 9.

13B
FALSE—Reference *E*, p. 9.

13C
FALSE—Reference *E*, p. 9.

13D
TRUE—The average life of a red blood cell is 120 days. Reference *E*, p. 9.

13E
FALSE—Reference *E*, p. 9.

14A
FALSE—Tactile nerves are found in the dermis. There are no nerve endings in the epidermis. Reference *K*, p. 163.

14B
FALSE—Sweat glands are not found in the epidermis, although their ducts pass through the epidermis to open onto the skin surface. Reference *K*, p. 163 (Fig. 11:2).

14C
FALSE—There are no blood vessels in the epidermis. Reference *K*, p. 162.

14D
TRUE—Keratin is found in the flat, dead cells on the outer surface of the epidermis. Reference *K*, p. 162.

14E
FALSE—Melanin is a brown pigment found in the germinative (deep) layer of the epidermis. Reference *K*, p. 164.

1.2 OSTEOLOGY

15 The condyle of the mandible articulates with the:

A. sphenoid bone.
B. occipital bone.
C. temporal bone.
D. parietal bone.
E. frontal bone.

16 The foramen spinosum transmits the:

A. mandibular nerve.
B. facial nerve.
C. internal carotid artery.
D. vertebral artery.
E. middle meningeal artery.

Answers overleaf

15A
FALSE—The sphenoid bone is situated in the centre of the base of the cranium. Reference *E*, pp. 32–34.

15B
FALSE—The occipital bone forms the posterior part of the base and vault of the cranium. Reference *E*, pp. 26 and 27.

15C
TRUE—The mandible articulates with the mandibular fossa on the zygomatic process of the squamous part of the temporal bone. Reference *E*, pp. 27 and 60.

15D
FALSE—The parietal bones are on either side of the midline and form part of the roof and sides of the cranium. Reference *E*, pp. 25 and 26.

15E
FALSE—The frontal bone forms the forehead, the roof of the orbits and part of the floor of the anterior cranial fossa. Reference *E*, pp. 24 and 25.

16A
FALSE—The mandibular branch of trigeminal nerve passes through the foramen ovale on the greater wing of sphenoid. Reference *D*, p. 157.

16B
FALSE—The facial nerve passes through the stylomastoid foramen. Reference *D*, p. 157.

16C
FALSE—The internal carotid artery passes through foramen lacerum. Reference *D*, p. 157.

16D
FALSE—The vertebral artery passes through the transverse foramina of the cervical vertebrae. Reference *D*, p. 163.

16E
TRUE—The middle meningeal artery passes through the foramen spinosum of sphenoid. Reference *D*, p. 157.

17 The spiral groove is on the:

A. femur.
B. humerus.
C. radius.
D. tibia.
E. ulna.

18 The obturator foramen is:

A. situated in the ilium.
B. enclosed by the ischium and the pubis.
C. the articulation for the head of the femur.
D. situated in the sacrum.
E. enclosed by the sacrum and the ilium.

Answers overleaf

17A
FALSE—Reference *E*, p. 154.

17B
TRUE—The spiral groove runs obliquely forwards and downwards over the lateral border of the humerus. Reference *E*, pp. 153 and 154.

17C
FALSE—Reference *E*, p. 154.

17D
FALSE—Reference *E*, p. 154.

17E
FALSE—Reference *E*, p. 154.

18A
FALSE—The ilium does not contain the obturator foramen. Reference *E*, p. 208.

18B
TRUE—The obturator foramen is enclosed by the body and ramus of the ischium and the superior and inferior rami of the pubis. Reference *E*, pp. 206 and 208.

18C
FALSE—The articulation for the head of femur is the acetabulum. Reference *E*, pp. 204, 205 and 209.

18D
FALSE—The sacrum contains the anterior and posterior intervertebral foramina, but not the obturator foramen. Reference *E*, pp. 92 and 93.

18E
FALSE—The sacrum and ilium form the sacroiliac joint. Reference *E*, pp. 216 and 217.

19 Which of the following is found in the proximal row of carpal bones?

A. Capitate.
B. Trapezium.
C. Triquetrum.
D. Trapezoid.
E. Hamate.

20 The foramina in the transverse processes of the cervical vertebrae transmit the:

A. internal carotid artery.
B. subclavian artery.
C. external carotid artery.
D. vertebral artery.
E. basilar artery.

Answers overleaf

19A
FALSE—Reference *E*, p. 178.

19B
FALSE—Reference *E*, p. 178.

19C
TRUE—From lateral to medial, the bones in the proximal row are the scaphoid, lunate, triquetrum and pisiform. Reference *E*, p. 178.

19D
FALSE—Reference *E*, p. 178.

19E
FALSE—Reference *E*, p. 178.

20A
FALSE—The internal carotid artery passes through the carotid canal of the temporal bone. Reference *G*, p. 149.

20B
FALSE—The subclavian artery passes through the thoracic inlet. Reference *H*, p. 58.

20C
FALSE—The external carotid artery lies on the pharyngeal wall. Reference *D*, p. 495.

20D
TRUE—The vertebral artery passes through the foramina in the transverse processes of the cervical vertebrae. Reference *G*, p. 106.

20E
FALSE—The basilar artery is on the undersurface of the brain (pons). Reference *D*, pp. 494 and 495.

21 The foramen ovale is found in the:

A. anterior cranial fossa.
B. orbital cavity.
C. middle cranial fossa.
D. nasal cavity.
E. posterior cranial fossa.

22 One feature of a lumbar vertebra is a:

A. mamillary process.
B. bifid spine.
C. transverse foramen.
D. costal facet.
E. heart-shaped body.

Answers overleaf

21A
FALSE—Reference *E*, pp. 21 and 22.

21B
FALSE—Reference *E*, pp. 21 and 22.

21C
TRUE—The foramen ovale is found in the anterior part of the floor of the middle cranial cavity. Reference *E*, pp. 21 and 22.

21D
FALSE—Reference *E*, pp. 21 and 22.

21E
FALSE—Reference *E*, pp. 21 and 22.

22A
TRUE—A mamillary process is one of the features of a lumbar vertebra. Reference *E*, p. 87.

22B
FALSE—A bifid spine is found on the 3rd to 6th cervical vertebrae. Reference *E*, pp. 73 and 74.

22C
FALSE—A transverse foramen is a feature of the cervical vertebrae. Reference *E*, pp. 73 and 74.

22D
FALSE—A costal facet is a feature of the thoracic vertebrae. Reference *E*, p. 82.

22E
FALSE—A heart-shaped body is a feature of a typical thoracic vertebra. Reference *E*, p. 81.

23 The conoid tubercle is a small prominence on the:

A. scapula.
B. humerus.
C. ribs.
D. clavicle.
E. ulna.

24 The external covering of a bone is the:

A. diaphysis.
B. endosteum.
C. epiphysis.
D. metaphysis.
E. periosteum.

Answers overleaf

23A
FALSE—The tubercles on the scapula are the supraglenoid and infraglenoid. Reference *E*, p. 135.

23B
FALSE—The humerus does not possess a feature known as the conoid tubercle. Reference *E*, pp. 152 and 153.

23C
FALSE—The 1st to 10th ribs possess a tubercle, but it is not described as conoid. Reference *E*, p. 119 and 122.

23D
TRUE—The conoid (cone-shaped) tubercle is on the inferior surface of the lateral part of the shaft of the clavicle. Reference *E*, pp. 145 and 146.

23E
FALSE—The ulna does not possess a feature known as the conoid tubercle. Reference *E*, pp. 173–175.

24A
FALSE—The diaphysis is the shaft of a long bone formed from the primary centre of ossification. Reference *E*, pp. 2 and 7.

24B
FALSE—The endosteum is vascular areolar tissue which lines the medullary cavity of the long bones. Reference *B*, p. 591.

24C
FALSE—The epiphysis is a secondary centre of ossification of a developing bone. Reference *E*, pp. 2 and 7.

24D
FALSE—The metaphysis is the actively growing area of the diaphysis immediately adjacent to the epiphyseal plate. Reference *E*, pp. 2 and 7.

24E
TRUE—The external covering of a bone, except the articular surface, is a thin vascular membrane called the periosteum. Reference *E*, pp. 5 and 7.

25 The lower end of the fibula is known as the:

A. medial malleolus.
B. lateral malleolus.
C. styloid process.
D. lateral condyle.
E. medial epicondyle.

26 The superior nasal concha is part of the:

A. ethmoid bone.
B. palatine bone.
C. zygomatic bone.
D. sphenoid bone.
E. frontal bone.

Answers overleaf

25A
FALSE—The medial malleolus is a downward prolongation of the medial surface of the lower extremity of tibia. Reference *E*, p. 259.

25B
TRUE—The lower end of the fibula is slightly expanded and projects downwards as the lateral malleolus. Reference *E*, p. 260.

25C
FALSE—The styloid process is the name given to the projection on the posterior surface of the head of the fibula. Reference *E*, p. 260.

25D
FALSE—The lateral condyle is on the upper extremity of the tibia. Reference *E*, pp. 256 and 258.

25E
FALSE—The medial epicondyle is a roughened prominence on the medial condyle of the lower extremity of the femur. Reference *E*, p. 239.

26A
TRUE—The superior nasal concha is part of the ethmoid bone and is on the lateral wall of the nasal cavity. Reference *E*, pp. 37 and 38.

26B
FALSE—Reference *E*, p. 37 (Fig. 2.25).

26C
FALSE—Reference *E*, p. 37 (Fig. 2.25).

26D
FALSE—Reference *E*, p. 37 (Fig. 2.25).

26E
FALSE—Reference *E*, p. 37 (Fig. 2.25).

27 The feature known as the linea aspera is found on the:

A. tibia.
B. femur.
C. ulna.
D. humerus.
E. fibula.

28 The crista galli is part of the:

A. frontal bone.
B. sphenoid bone.
C. palatine bone.
D. lacrimal bone.
E. ethmoid bone.

Answers overleaf

27A
FALSE—The oblique ridge on the posterior surface of the upper extremity of the tibia is called the soleal line. Reference *E*, pp. 257 (Fig. 8.23) and 259.

27B
TRUE—The linea aspera is a longitudinal bony ridge on the posterior aspect of the femur. Reference *E*, p. 238.

27C
FALSE—Reference *E*, p. 238.

27D
FALSE—Reference *E*, p. 238.

27E
FALSE—Reference *E*, p. 238.

28A
FALSE—Reference *E*, p. 35.

28B
FALSE—Reference *E*, p. 35.

28C
FALSE—Reference *E*, p. 35.

28D
FALSE—Reference *E*, p. 35.

28E
TRUE—The projection above the horizontal plate of the ethmoid bone is called the crista galli. Reference *E*, pp. 34 (Figs. 2.21 and 2.22) and 35.

1.3 ARTHROLOGY

29 The term 'inversion' refers to one of the movements of the:

A. elbow.
B. foot.
C. hand.
D. hip.
E. shoulder.

30 The ligament around the head of the radius is the:

A. ligamentum teres.
B. collateral ligament.
C. ulnar ligament.
D. annular ligament.
E. brachial ligament.

Answers overleaf

29A
FALSE—The elbow is a synovial hinge joint, and the only movement possible is flexion or extension. Reference *E*, p. 164.

29B
TRUE—Inversion, a turning inward, occurs at the anterior and posterior subtalar joints and the calcaneocuboid joint of the foot. Reference *E*, pp. 285–289.

29C
FALSE—Inward rotation of the hand is called pronation and occurs at the superior radioulnar joint. Reference *E*, p. 169.

29D
FALSE—Inward rotation of the hip joint is called medial rotation. Reference *E*, p. 228.

29E
FALSE—Inward movement at the shoulder is also called medial rotation. Reference *E*, p. 141.

30A
FALSE—The ligamentum teres is attached to the fovea of the femoral head and the acetabular rim. Reference *E*, p. 227.

30B
FALSE—Collateral ligaments are present in many joints. One associated with the elbow arises from the lateral epicondyle of the humerus and attaches to the lateral side of the annular ligament. Reference *E*, p. 163.

30C
FALSE—The ulnar ligament passes from the tip of the styloid process of the ulna and is attached to the triquetral and pisiform bones. Reference *E*, p. 190.

30D
TRUE—The annular ligament is a strong band which encircles the head of the radius, being attached to the anterior and posterior margins of the radial notch of the ulna. Reference *E*, p. 169.

30E
FALSE—The brachial ligament can refer to one of the two collateral ligaments of the elbow joint. Reference *E*, p. 163.

31 The coronal suture separates the:

A. left and right parietal bones.
B. parietal and frontal bones.
C. temporal and frontal bones.
D. parietal and temporal bones.
E. temporal and occipital bones.

32 The bone in the carpus having only one articular facet is the:

A. scaphoid.
B. hamate.
C. pisiform
D. triquetrum.
E. trapezoid.

Answers overleaf

31A
FALSE—The suture between the left and right parietal bones is the sagittal suture. Reference *E*, p. 25.

31B
TRUE—The coronal suture is between the parietal and frontal bones. Reference *E*, p. 25.

31C
FALSE—The temporal and frontal bones do not articulate with each other. Reference *E*, p. 15 (Fig. 2.5).

31D
FALSE—The suture between the parietal and temporal bones is part of the squamous suture. Reference *H*, p. 8.

31E
FALSE—The suture between the temporal and occipital bones is the occipitomastoid suture. Reference *E*, p. 15 (Fig. 2.5).

32A
FALSE—The scaphoid articulates with trapezium, trapezoid, capitate, lunate and radius. Reference *E*, p. 180.

32B
FALSE—The hamate articulates with the 4th and 5th metacarpal bones, capitate, triquetrum and lunate. Reference *E*, p. 180 (Fig. 6.26).

32C
TRUE—The pisiform has only one articulation with the triquetrum. Reference *E*, p. 179 (Fig. 6.25) and 181.

32D
FALSE—The triquetrum articulates with hamate, lunate and pisiform. Reference *E*, p. 180 (Fig. 6.26).

32E
FALSE—The trapezoid articulates with the 2nd metacarpal bone, trapezium, capitate and scaphoid. Reference *E*, p. 181.

33 Which of the following articular surfaces is involved in the radiocarpal (wrist) joint?

A. The proximal surface of pisiform.
B. The head of ulna.
C. The distal surface of scaphoid.
D. The proximal surface of lunate.
E. The head of radius.

34 The lambdoid suture is located between the:

A. sphenoid and temporal bones.
B. occipital and frontal bones.
C. parietal and occipital bones.
D. frontal and parietal bones.
E. sphenoid and parietal bones.

Answers overleaf

33A
FALSE—The pisiform only articulates with triquetrum. Reference *E*, p. 181.

33B
FALSE—The head of ulna is separated from the carpal bones by a triangular fibrocartilaginous articular disc. Reference *E*, p. 190.

33C
FALSE—The distal surface of scaphoid articulates with trapezoid and trapezium. Reference *E*, p. 180 (Fig. 6.26).

33D
TRUE—The proximal surface of lunate is one of the articular surfaces involved in the formation of the wrist joint. Reference *E*, p. 190.

33E
FALSE—The head of radius is one of the articular surfaces of the elbow joint. Reference *E*, p. 163.

34A
FALSE—The articulation of the sphenoid and temporal bones is called the sphenosquamosal suture. Reference *G*, p. 146.

34B
FALSE—The occipital and frontal bones do not form an articulation. Reference *G*, p. 131 (Fig. 10.2).

34C
TRUE—Part of the lambdoid suture is located between the parietal and occipital bones. Reference *G*, pp. 141 (Fig. 10.10) and 144.

34D
FALSE—The articulation of the frontal and parietal bones forms part of the coronal suture. Reference *G*, pp. 141 (Fig. 10.10) and 153.

34E
FALSE—The articulation of the sphenoid and parietal bones is called the sphenoparietal suture. Reference *B*, p. 1640.

35 The head of a typical rib articulates with the:

A. costal cartilages.
B. sternum.
C. vertebral bodies.
D. transverse processes.
E. pedicles.

36 Which of the following terms describe the manubriosternal joint?

A. Gomphosis.
B. Synovial joint.
C. Synchondrosis.
D. Symphysis.
E. Suture.

Answers overleaf

35A
FALSE—The anterior end of a typical rib articulates with the costal cartilages, the head being part of the posterior end. Reference *E*, pp. 119 and 128.

35B
FALSE—The sternum has articular facets for the clavicles and 1st to 7th costal cartilages. Reference *E*, pp. 113–115 (Figs 4.3 and 4.4).

35C
TRUE—The head (part of the posterior end) of a typical rib articulates with adjacent vertebral bodies. Reference *E*, pp. 81, 82 (Fig. 3.18) and 119.

35D
FALSE—The tubercle of the rib articulates with the transverse process. Reference *E*, p. 119.

35E
FALSE—The pedicle does not articulate with the head of a typical rib. Reference *E*, p. 81.

36A
FALSE—A gomphosis is a type of fibrous joint found between the teeth and jaw. Reference *E*, p. 10.

36B
FALSE—The manubriosternal joint does not contain a synovial membrane. Reference *E*, pp. 10–11 and 128.

36C
FALSE—A synchondrosis is a type of cartilaginous joint found between the sternal segments. Reference *E*, p. 10.

36D
TRUE—The manubriosternal joint is a symphysis, a type of cartilaginous joint. Reference *E*, p. 10 and 128.

36E
FALSE—A suture is a fibrous joint found between the bones of the skull. Reference *E*, p. 10.

37 Deposition of uric acid salts in a joint causes:

A. rickets.
B. gout.
C. ankylosis.
D. recurrent dislocation.
E. osteoporosis.

38 Which of the following terms describes the sacroiliac joint?

A. Cartilaginous.
B. Saddle.
C. Fibrous.
D. Condylar.
E. Plane (gliding).

Answers overleaf

37A
FALSE—Rickets is a disorder of infancy and childhood caused by vitamin D deficiency. Reference *I*, p. 238.

37B
TRUE—Gout is characterised by deposition of uric acid salts in and around joints. Reference *I*, p. 260.

37C
FALSE—Ankylosis is the union of opposing joint surfaces by fibrous tissue or newly formed bone. Reference *I*, p. 247.

37D
FALSE—Recurrent dislocation is where dislocation repeatedly recurs after reduction. Reference *B*, p. 529.

37E
FALSE—Osteoporosis is where bones contain less bone tissue than normal bones do. Reference *I*, p. 238.

38A
FALSE—The sacroiliac joint is classified as a synovial joint. Reference *E*, p. 216.

38B
FALSE—An example of a saddle joint is the 1st carpometacarpal joint. Reference *E*, pp. 11 and 199.

38C
FALSE—Fibrous joints do not allow any movement and the sacroiliac joint is synovial. Reference *E*, pp. 10 and 216.

38D
FALSE—An example of a condylar joint is the temporomandibular joint. Reference *E*, pp. 11 and 60.

38E
TRUE—The sacroiliac joint is a synovial joint and classified as a plane (gliding) joint. Reference *E*, pp. 11 and 216.

1.4 MYOLOGY

39 Which of the following is the name for the heart muscle?

A. Pericardium.
B. Myometrium.
C. Endocardium.
D. Tunica media.
E. Myocardium.

40 The muscle arising from the anterior surface of the scapula is the:

A. subscapularis.
B. supraspinatus.
C. infraspinatus.
D. teres minor.
E. teres major.

Answers overleaf

39A
FALSE—The pericardium is the serous membrane which encloses the heart. Reference *D*, p. 460.

39B
FALSE—The myometrium is the middle layer of the uterus consisting of smooth muscle fibres. Reference *D*, p. 724.

39C
FALSE—The endocardium is a thin epithelial layer lining the inside of the myocardium. Reference *D*, p. 461.

39D
FALSE—The tunica media is the middle coat of the artery wall consisting of elastic and smooth muscle fibres. Reference *D*, p. 486.

39E
TRUE—The myocardium is the middle layer of the heart wall, and contains the heart muscle. Reference *D*, p. 461.

40A
TRUE—The subscapularis muscle originates from the anterior (costal) surface of the scapula. Reference *E*, pp. 132 and 141.

40B
FALSE—The supraspinatus muscle originates from the supraspinous fossa on the posterior (dorsal) surface of the scapula. Reference *E*, pp. 133 and 141.

40C
FALSE—The infraspinatus muscle originates from the infraspinous fossa on the posterior (dorsal) surface of the scapula.
Reference *E*, pp. 133 and 141.

40D
FALSE—The teres minor muscle originates from the lateral border of the scapula. Reference *E*, p. 136 (Fig. 5.5).

40E
FALSE—The teres major muscle originates from the lateral part of the inferior angle. Reference *E*, pp. 136 (Fig. 5.5) and 142.

41 The crura of the diaphragm originate from the:

A. xiphoid process of the sternum.
B. fascia of the posterior abdominal wall.
C. 1st–3rd lumbar vertebrae.
D. lower 6 pairs of ribs.
E. costal cartilages.

42 The infraspinatus muscle is inserted into the humerus at the:

A. greater tuberosity.
B. bicipital groove.
C. surgical neck.
D. lesser tuberosity.
E. anatomical neck.

Answers overleaf

41A
FALSE—The anterior muscle fibres of the diaphragm originate from the posterior surface of the xiphoid process. Reference *E*, p. 128.

41B
FALSE—The fascia of the posterior abdominal wall supports the parietal peritoneum. Reference *D*, p. 598.

41C
TRUE—The right crus of the diaphragm arises from the upper three lumbar vertebrae; the left crus arises from the upper two lumbar vertebrae. Reference *E*, p. 128.

41D
FALSE—The lateral muscle fibres of the diaphragm originate from the lower six pairs of ribs. Reference *E*, p. 128.

41E
FALSE—The lateral muscle fibres of the diaphragm originate from the lower six costal cartilages. Reference *E*, p. 128.

42A
TRUE—The infraspinatus muscle is inserted into the middle of the three areas for muscle attachment on the greater tuberosity of humerus. Reference *E*, pp. 141 and 152.

42B
FALSE—The pectoralis major, latissimus dorsi and teres major muscles are inserted into the lips of the bicipital groove. Reference *E*, pp. 142 and 152.

42C
FALSE—The surgical neck is a constricted portion just distal to the greater and lesser tuberosity, named because of its liability to fracture. Reference *D*, p. 178.

42D
FALSE—The subscapularis muscle is inserted into the lesser tuberosity. Reference *E*, pp. 141 and 152.

42E
FALSE—The anatomical neck separates the head of humerus from the shaft and gives attachment to the capsular ligament of the shoulder joint. Reference *E*, p. 152.

43 Extension of the elbow joint is produced by which of the following muscles?

A. Biceps brachii.
B. Brachialis.
C. Triceps.
D. Deltoid.
E. Brachioradialis.

44 Which of the following muscles is superficial on the anterior abdominal wall?

A. Rectus abdominis.
B. Sacrospinalis.
C. Quadratus lumborum.
D. Psoas major.
E. Pectoralis major.

Answers overleaf

43A
FALSE—The biceps brachii muscle is a flexor of the elbow joint. Reference *E*, p. 164.

43B
FALSE—The brachialis muscle assists the biceps brachii in flexing the elbow joint. Reference *E*, p. 164.

43C
TRUE—The triceps muscle is an extensor of the elbow joint. Reference *E*, p. 164.

43D
FALSE—The deltoid muscle extends, flexes and abducts the shoulder joint. Reference *E*, p. 142.

43E
FALSE—The brachioradialis muscle flexes the elbow joint. Reference *E*, p. 165.

44A
TRUE—The rectus abdominis muscle lies superficial on the anterior abdominal wall, forming visible ridges on either side of the midline. Reference *J*, pp. 67, 68 and 69 (Fig. 31).

44B
FALSE—The sacrospinalis muscle lies superficial on the posterior abdominal wall. Reference *J*, pp. 69 and 70 (Fig. 32).

44C
FALSE—The quadratus lumborum lies lateral to sacrospinalis on the posterior abdominal wall. Reference *J*, p. 70 (Fig. 32).

44D
FALSE—The psoas major muscle lies anterior to the transverse processes of the lumbar vertebrae. Reference *J*, p. 70 (Fig. 32).

44E
FALSE—The pectoralis major muscle covers the anterior and lateral chest walls. Reference *J*, p. 56.

45 The long head of biceps arises from the:

A. coracoid process of the scapula.
B. greater tuberosity of the humerus.
C. lesser tuberosity of the humerus.
D. supraglenoid tubercle.
E. labrum glenoidale.

Answers overleaf

45A
FALSE—The short head of biceps brachii and the coracobrachialis arise from the coracoid process of the scapula. Reference *E*, pp. 136 (Fig. 5.4), 142 and 164.

45B
FALSE—The greater tuberosity provides attachment for supraspinatus, infraspinatus and teres minor, which arise from the scapula. Reference *E*, pp. 141 and 152.

45C
FALSE—The lesser tuberosity gives attachment to the subscapularis muscle which arises from the scapula. Reference *E*, pp. 136 (Fig. 5.4), 141 and 152.

45D
TRUE—The long head of biceps arises from the supraglenoid tubercle of scapula. Reference *E*, pp. 135 and 164.

45E
FALSE—The labrum glenoidale is a fibrocartilaginous rim attached to the periphery of the glenoid cavity and deepens the joint cavity. Reference *E*, pp. 135 and 140 (Fig. 5.8).

1.5 ANGIOLOGY

46 The caecum derives its blood supply from the:

A. inferior mesenteric artery.
B. right common iliac artery.
C. coeliac trunk.
D. right internal iliac artery.
E. superior mesenteric artery.

47 The left ovarian/testicular (gonadal) vein drains directly into the:

A. left renal vein.
B. inferior vena cava.
C. left internal iliac vein.
D. inferior mesenteric vein.
E. left inferior vesicular vein.

Answers overleaf

46A

FALSE—The inferior mesenteric artery supplies the distal half of the large intestine and part of the rectum. Reference *K*, pp. 76 and 77 (Fig. 5:37).

46B

FALSE—The right common iliac artery divides into the internal and external iliac arteries to supply the pelvic organs and the right lower limb. Reference *K*, pp. 76 (Fig. 5:35) and 78.

46C

FALSE—The coeliac trunk is 1.25 cm long and divides into the left gastric, splenic and common hepatic arteries. Reference *K*, pp. 76 and 77 (Fig. 5:36).

46D

FALSE—The right internal iliac artery supplies organs within the pelvic cavity. Reference *K*, pp. 76 (Fig. 5:35), 78 and 79.

46E

TRUE—The superior mesenteric artery supplies the whole of the small intestine and the proximal half of the large intestine (including the caecum). Reference *K*, pp. 76 and 77 (Fig. 5:37).

47A

TRUE—The left gonadal vein drains directly into the left renal vein. Reference *L*, p. 153.

47B

FALSE—The right gonadal vein drains directly into the inferior vena cava. Reference *L*, p. 153.

47C

FALSE—The left internal iliac vein receives blood from the organs within the pelvic cavity, but not the left gonadal vein. Reference *L*, p. 200.

47D

FALSE—The inferior mesenteric vein returns the venous blood from the rectum, descending and pelvic colon. Reference *K*, p. 78 (Fig. 5:38).

47E

FALSE—The left inferior vesicular vein receives blood from the structures around the base of the bladder. Reference *L*, p. 200.

48 The vertebral artery passes through the:

A. intervertebral foramina.
B. obturator foramen.
C. transverse foramina.
D. vertebral foramina.
E. foramen spinosum.

49 The coronary sinus drains into the:

A. superior vena cava.
B. right atrium.
C. left ventricle.
D. pulmonary vein.
E. inferior vena cava.

Answers overleaf

48A
FALSE—The intervertebral foramina lie between the pedicles of adjacent vertebrae and transmit the spinal nerves and vessels. Reference *E*, p. 73.

48B
FALSE—The obturator foramen of the pelvic bones transmits the obturator vessels and nerve from the pelvis to the thigh. Reference *E*, p. 208.

48C
TRUE—The transverse foramina of the transverse processes of the cervical vertebrae allow passage of the vertebral vessels. Reference *E*, p. 74.

48D
FALSE—The vertebral foramina contains the spinal cord, meninges and associated vessels. Reference *E*, p. 71.

48E
FALSE—The foramen spinosum transmits the middle meningeal artery. Reference *E*, p. 22.

49A
FALSE—The superior vena cava drains the venous blood from the head, neck and upper limb. Reference *K*, p. 73 (Fig. 5:30).

49B
TRUE—The venous return from the heart is by the coronary sinus which drains into the right atrium. Reference *K*, p. 62.

49C
FALSE—The left ventricle is concerned only with oxygenated blood. Reference *K*, p. 62.

49D
FALSE—The pulmonary veins carry oxygenated blood and empty into the left atrium. Reference *K*, p. 61.

49E
FALSE—The inferior vena cava receives blood from all parts of the body below the diaphragm and conveys it to the right atrium. Reference *K*, p. 76.

50 The first half of the large intestine receives blood from the:

A. left gastric artery.
B. gastroepiploic artery.
C. portal vein.
D. superior mesenteric artery.
E. inferior mesenteric artery.

51 The splenic artery is a branch of the:

A. coeliac axis.
B. superior mesenteric artery.
C. left gastric artery.
D. inferior phrenic artery.
E. hepatic artery.

Answers overleaf

50A
FALSE—The left gastric artery, a branch of the coeliac artery, supplies blood to the lesser curvature of the stomach. Reference *K*, pp. 76 and 77 (Fig. 5:36).

50B
FALSE—The gastroepiploic arteries supply the greater curvature of the stomach and the greater omentum. Reference *K*, p. 77 (Fig. 5:36).

50C
FALSE—The portal vein drains the abdominal and the majority of the pelvic parts of the alimentary canal. Reference *K*, p. 78 (Fig. 5:38).

50D
TRUE—The superior mesenteric artery supplies the proximal half of the large intestine and the whole of the small intestine. Reference *K*, pp. 76 and 77 (Fig. 5:37).

50E
FALSE—The inferior mesenteric artery supplies the distal half of the large intestine and part of the rectum. Reference *K*, pp. 76 and 77 (Fig. 5:37).

51A
TRUE—The coeliac axis has three main branches; the left gastric common hepatic and splenic arteries. Reference *K*, pp. 76 and 77 (Fig. 5:36).

51B
FALSE—The superior mesenteric artery does not have any major named branches. Reference *K*, p. 76.

51C
FALSE—The left gastric artery is a branch of the coeliac artery. Reference *K*, pp. 76 and 77 (Fig. 5:36).

51D
FALSE—The inferior phrenic artery is a branch of the abdominal aorta and supplies the diaphragm. Reference *K*, p. 76 (Fig. 5:35).

51E
FALSE—The hepatic artery is a branch of the coeliac artery, supplying the liver and gall bladder and parts of the stomach, duodenum and pancreas. Reference *K*, pp. 76 and 77 (Fig. 5:36).

52 Blood flows from the subclavian artery into the:

A. brachial artery.
B. maxillary artery.
C. brachiocephalic artery.
D. axillary artery.
E. occipital artery.

53 The inferior vena cava commences at the level of which of the following vertebrae?

A. 6th thoracic.
B. 8th thoracic.
C. 12th thoracic.
D. 2nd lumbar.
E. 5th lumbar.

Answers overleaf

52A
FALSE—The brachial artery is a continuation of the axillary artery and lies in the upper arm. Reference *K*, pp. 73 and 74 (Fig. 5:31).

52B
FALSE—The maxillary artery is a branch of the external carotid artery in the region of the temporomandibular joint. Reference *K*, p. 71 (Fig. 5:24).

52C
FALSE—The brachiocephalic artery is the first branch of the arch of the aorta and branches into the right common carotid and right subclavian arteries. Reference *K*, pp. 67 and 70 (Fig. 5.23).

52D
TRUE—The subclavian artery continues as the axillary artery after passing over the first rib and enters the axilla. Reference *K*, pp. 73 and 74 (Fig. 5:31).

52E
FALSE—The occipital artery is a branch of the external carotid artery and supplies the posterior part of the scalp. Reference *K*, p. 71 (Fig. 5:24).

53A
FALSE—Reference *K*, p. 76.

53B
FALSE—Reference *K*, p. 76.

53C
FALSE—The level of the 12th thoracic vertebra is the level of commencement of the abdominal aorta. Reference *K*, p. 76.

53D
FALSE—The level of the 2nd lumbar vertebra is the level of formation of the portal vein. Reference *J*, pp. 79 (Fig. 40) and 84.

53E
TRUE—The inferior vena cava commences at the level of the 5th lumbar vertebra by the junction of the right and left common iliac veins. Reference *K*, p. 76.

54 Blood from the superior vena cava drains directly into the:

A. left ventricle.
B. pulmonary trunk.
C. right atrium.
D. pulmonary veins.
E. great cardiac vein.

55 The impulses for the contraction of the heart muscle normally originate in the:

A. atrioventricular bundle.
B. fibres of Purkinje.
C. sinoatrial node.
D. atrioventricular node.
E. bundle of His.

Answers overleaf

54A
FALSE—Blood entering the left ventricle is from the left atrium. Reference *K*, p. 61.

54B
FALSE—Blood entering the pulmonary trunk is from the right ventricle. Reference *K*, p. 61.

54C
TRUE—Blood from the superior vena cava drains directly into the right atrium. Reference *K*, p. 61.

54D
FALSE—The blood entering the pulmonary veins is from the lungs. Reference *K*, p. 61.

54E
FALSE—The great cardiac vein drains blood from the left side of the heart. Reference *L*, pp. 40 and 41 (Fig. 55).

55A
FALSE—The atrioventricular bundle, found in the septum between the right and left ventricles, is part of the conducting system but does not initiate contraction. Reference *K*, pp. 62 (Fig. 5:13) and 63.

55B
FALSE—The fibres of Purkinje convey the impulses to the myocardium of the ventricles. Reference *K*, pp. 62 (Fig. 5:13) and 63.

55C
TRUE—The sinoatrial node in the wall of the right atrium is where the impulses are normally initiated. Reference *K*, p. 62 (Fig. 5:13).

55D
FALSE—The atrioventricular node in the atrial septum is normally stimulated by the contraction of the atrial myocardium. Reference *K*, pp. 62 (Fig. 5:13) and 63.

55E
FALSE—The Bundle of His is an alternative name for the atrioventricular bundle. Reference *K*, p. 63.

56 The cardiac valve situated between the left atrium and the left ventricle is the:

A. tricuspid valve.
B. aortic valve.
C. mitral valve.
D. coronary valve.
E. pulmonary valve.

57 The superior mesenteric artery arises directly from the:

A. coeliac axis.
B. hepatic artery.
C. abdominal aorta.
D. splenic artery.
E. left gastric artery.

Answers overleaf

56A
FALSE—The tricuspid valve is another name for the right atrioventricular valve. Reference *K*, pp. 60 and 61 (Fig. 5:9).

56B
FALSE—The aortic valve is situated between the left ventricle and the ascending aorta. Reference *K*, pp. 61 (Fig. 5:9) and 62.

56C
TRUE—The mitral valve is situated between the left atrium and the left ventricle. Reference *K*, pp. 60 and 61 (Fig. 5:9).

56D
FALSE—The coronary valve is situated between the coronary sinus and the right atrium. Reference *L*, pp. 41 and 42 (Fig. 57).

56E
FALSE—The pulmonary valve is situated between the right ventricle and the pulmonary artery *K*, p. 61 (Fig. 5:9).

57A
FALSE—The coeliac axis has three main branches; the left gastric common hepatic and splenic arteries. Reference *K*, pp. 76 and 77 (Fig. 5:36).

57B
FALSE—The branches of the hepatic artery are the right gastric and right and left hepatic arteries. Reference *L*, p. 109.

57C
TRUE—The superior mesenteric artery arises directly from the abdominal aorta in the midline 1 cm below the coeliac artery. Reference *K*, p. 76 (Fig. 5:35).

57D
FALSE—The only major branch of the splenic artery is the left gastroepiploic artery. Reference *K*, p. 77 (Fig. 5:36).

57E
FALSE—The left gastric artery has small gastric and ascending oesophageal branches only. Reference *L*, p. 109.

58 Oxygenated blood, during ventricular systole, flows:

A. through the pulmonary valve.
B. into the right ventricle.
C. through the mitral valve.
D. into the right atrium.
E. through the aortic valve.

59 The rate of blood flow through the kidneys is:

A. 0.12 ml/min.
B. 1.2 ml/min.
C. 12 ml/min.
D. 120 ml/min.
E. 1200 ml/min.

Answers overleaf

58A
FALSE—Deoxygenated blood flows through the pulmonary valve during ventricular systole. Reference *K*, p. 61.

58B
FALSE—Deoxygenated blood flows into the right ventricle during atrial systole. Reference *K*, pp. 61 and 63.

58C
FALSE—During ventricular systole, the mitral (left atrioventricular) valve is closed. Reference *K*, pp. 60 and 64.

58D
FALSE—Deoxygenated blood flows into the right atrium during diastole. Reference *K*, pp. 61 and 63.

58E
TRUE—During ventricular systole, oxygenated blood flows through the aortic valve. Reference *K*, pp. 61, 62 and 63.

59A
FALSE—The figure is near to the minimum (obligatory) volume of urine produced. Reference *F*, p. 136.

59B
FALSE—This figure is near to that of normal urine production. Reference *F*, p. 136.

59C
FALSE—Reference *F*, p. 135.

59D
FALSE—This is the volume of filtrate produced per minute and termed the glomerular filtration rate. Reference *F*, pp. 135 and 136 (Fig. 140).

59E
TRUE—The rate of blood flow through the kidneys is 1200 ml/min. Reference *F*, p. 135.

1.6 RETICULO-ENDOTHELIAL SYSTEM

60 Which of the following statements applies to a lymph node?

A. Produces lymphocytes.
B. Secretes lymphatic fluid.
C. Absorbs water.
D. Produces lymphoid hormones.
E. Absorbs serum.

61 The thoracic duct returns the lymph to the circulation by:

A. re-absorption by the tissues.
B. re-entry into the blood capillaries.
C. entry into the superior vena cava.
D. the portal venous system.
E. the left subclavian vein.

Answers overleaf

60A

TRUE—Lymphocytes are produced within the germinal follicles found in a lymph node. Reference *M*, p. 770.

60B

FALSE—Lymph is produced by tissue fluid passing into lymphatic vessels. Reference *M*, p. 54.

60C

FALSE—Water absorption is not a function of a lymph node. Reference *K*, p. 87.

60D

FALSE—Hormone production is not a function of a lymph node. Reference *M*, p. 773.

60E

FALSE—Serum is blood plasma from which the fibrinogen has been removed. Reference *K*, p. 42.

61A

FALSE—Lymph is returned to the circulation by the thoracic duct opening into the left subclavian vein near its junction with the left internal jugular vein. Reference *K*, p. 85 (Fig. 6:4).

61B

FALSE—Reference *K*, p. 85.

61C

FALSE—Reference *K*, p. 85.

61D

FALSE—The portal venous system drains the abdominal part of the digestive tract and the spleen, and conveys the blood to the liver. Reference *K*, pp. 76 and 78 (Fig. 5:38).

61E

TRUE—The thoracic duct returns the lymph via the left subclavian vein near its junction with the left internal jugular vein. Reference *K*, p. 85 (Fig. 6:4).

62 The group of nodes receiving lymph from the stomach is the:

A. superior mesenteric.
B. external iliac.
C. coeliac.
D. ileocolic.
E. lateral aortic.

63 The first group of nodes receiving lymph from the sigmoid colon is the:

A. left colic.
B. ileocolic.
C. middle colic.
D. right colic.
E. paracolic.

Answers overleaf

62A
FALSE—The superior mesenteric nodes receive lymph from the small and proximal part of the large intestine. Reference *M*, p. 794.

62B
FALSE—The external iliac nodes receive lymph from part of the abdominal wall, the thigh area and some of the pelvic viscera. Reference *M*, p. 796.

62C
TRUE—The coeliac nodes are the terminal group receiving lymph from the stomach. Reference *M*, p. 793.

62D
FALSE—The ileocolic nodes receive lymph from the terminal ileum, caecum and vermiform appendix. Reference *M*, p. 795 (Fig. 6.170).

62E
FALSE—The lateral aortic nodes receive lymph from the viscera and other structures supplied by the lateral and dorsal branches of the aorta. Reference *M*, p. 793.

63A
TRUE—Lymph from the sigmoid colon passes first to the small nodes associated with the left colic arteries and then to the preaortic nodes near the inferior mesenteric artery. Reference *M*, p. 795.

63B
FALSE—The ileocolic nodes receive lymph from the terminal ileum, caecum and vermiform appendix. Reference *M*, p. 795 (Fig. 6.170).

63C
FALSE—The middle colic nodes are a part of the intermediate colic nodes and receive lymph from parts of the ascending and transverse colon. Reference *M*, p. 795.

63D
FALSE—The right colic nodes receive lymph from parts of the ascending and transverse colon. Reference *M*, p. 795.

63E
FALSE—The paracolic nodes receive lymph from the ascending and descending colon. Reference *M*, p. 795.

64 The thoracic duct commences at the level of the:

A. upper border of 4th thoracic vertebra.
B. upper border of 6th thoracic vertebra.
C. lower border of 9th thoracic vertebra.
D. lower border of 12th thoracic vertebra.
E. lower border of 2nd lumbar vertebra.

Answers overleaf

64A

FALSE—The thoracic duct commences in the abdominal cavity. Reference *M*, p. 784.

64B

FALSE—The thoracic duct is starting to incline to the left side of the midline at this point. Reference *M*, p. 784.

64C

FALSE—The thoracic duct commences in the abdominal cavity. Reference *M*, p. 784.

64D

TRUE—The thoracic duct begins at the upper end of the cisterna chyli near the lower border of the 12th thoracic vertebra. Reference *M*, p. 784.

64E

FALSE—The cisterna chyli commences at the level of the 2nd lumbar vertebra. Reference *M*, p. 785.

1.7 NEUROLOGY (GENERAL)

65 The interventricular foramen (foramen of Munro) connects the:

A. lateral and fourth ventricles.
B. lateral and third ventricles.
C. third and fourth ventricles.
D. fourth ventricle and the spinal cord.
E. fourth ventricle and basal cistern.

66 The pons is situated:

A. above the midbrain.
B. below the medulla oblongata.
C. below the midbrain.
D. behind the medulla oblongata.
E. behind the cerebellum.

Answers overleaf

65A

FALSE—The lateral and fourth ventricles are not in direct communication. Reference *K*, p. 173 (Fig. 12:9).

65B

TRUE—The interventricular foramen connects the lateral to the third ventricle. Reference *K*, p. 173.

65C

FALSE—The third and fourth ventricles are connected by the aqueduct of the midbrain (aqueduct of Sylvius). Reference *K*, p. 173.

65D

FALSE—The fourth ventricle and the spinal cord communicate via the central canal. Reference *K*, p. 173.

65E

FALSE—The fourth ventricles and the basal cistern are not in direct communication. Reference *N*, p. 39 (Plate 18).

66A

FALSE—The midbrain is above the pons. Reference *O*, p. 263 (Fig. 9–12).

66B

FALSE—The medulla oblongata is below the pons. Reference *O*, p. 263 (Fig. 9–12).

66C

TRUE—The pons is situated below the midbrain. Reference *O*, p. 263 (Fig. 9–12).

66D

FALSE—The pons is above the medulla oblongata. Reference *O*, p. 263 (Fig. 9–12).

66E

FALSE—The pons is in front of the cerebellum. Reference *O*, p. 263 (Fig. 9–12).

67 In the adult, the spinal cord usually ends at the level of the:

A. 1st lumbar vertebra.
B. 3rd lumbar vertebra.
C. 5th lumbar vertebra.
D. 1st sacral segment.
E. 3rd sacral segment.

68 The nerve supply to the oesophagus is from the:

A. vagus.
B. hypoglossal nerve.
C. glossopharyngeal nerve.
D. thoracic nerve.
E. phrenic nerve.

Answers overleaf

67A

TRUE—The spinal cord ends at the level of the lower border of the 1st lumbar vertebra or the upper level of the 2nd lumbar vertebra. Reference *P*, pp. 395 and 397 (Fig. 236).

67B

FALSE—The cord reaches the level of the 3rd lumbar vertebra at birth. Reference *P*, p. 396 (Fig. 235).

67C

FALSE—Reference *P*, pp. 395 and 397 (Fig. 236).

67D

FALSE—Reference *P*, pp. 395 and 397 (Fig. 236).

67E

FALSE—This is the approximate limit of the dura mater within the vertebral canal. Reference *P*, p. 397 (Fig. 236).

68A

TRUE—The vagus supplies the oesophagus with motor fibres for the smooth muscle and secretory glands and receives sensory fibres from the epithelial lining of the oesophagus. Reference *P*, p. 449.

68B

FALSE—The hypoglossal nerve supplies the intrinsic and extrinsic muscles of the tongue. Reference *P*, p. 452.

68C

FALSE—The glossopharyngeal nerve contains sensory fibres for the pharynx and posterior third of the tongue and motor fibres for the muscles of the pharynx and parotid gland. Reference *P*, p. 448.

68D

FALSE—The thoracic nerves supply the intercostal muscles and anterior and posterior abdominal walls. Reference *P*, pp. 14 and 15 (Fig. 9).

68E

FALSE—The phrenic nerve supplies the diaphragm and receives sensory fibres from the central part of the diaphragm. Reference *P*, pp. 16 and 17.

69 An inflammatory condition affecting the brain cortex is known as:

A. meningitis.
B. haemangioma.
C. encephalitis.
D. elephantiasis.
E. glioma.

70 The arachnoid mater is located between the:

A. dura mater and pia mater.
B. skull vault and dura mater.
C. cerebral cortex and pia mater.
D. falx cerebri and dura mater.
E. basal ganglia and pia mater.

Answers overleaf

69A
FALSE—Meningitis is inflammation of the meninges. Reference *I*, p. 277.

69B
FALSE—Haemangioma is a tumour of vascular tissue. Reference *I*, pp. 230 and 231.

69C
TRUE—Encephalitis is inflammation of brain tissue. Reference *I*, p. 277.

69D
FALSE—Elephantiasis is a blockage of lymphatic channels due to a nematode infestation. Reference *I*, p. 313.

69E
FALSE—Glioma is a malignant tumour arising from the supportive connective tissue of the central nervous system. Reference *I*, p. 280.

70A
TRUE—The arachnoid mater is a delicate serous membrane situated between the dura mater and pia mater. Reference *K*, pp. 172 (Fig. 12:7) and 173.

70B
FALSE—The outer layer of the dura mater lines the inner surface of the skull vault and takes the place of periosteum. Reference *K*, pp. 171 and 172 (Fig. 12:7).

70C
FALSE—The pia mater is a vascular membrane that closely invests the brain. Reference *K*, pp. 172 (Fig. 12:7) and 173.

70D
FALSE—The falx cerebri is formed by the inner layer of the dura mater and the space between the two layers of the dura mater forms a venous sinus. Reference *K*, pp. 171 and 172 (Fig 12:7).

70E
FALSE—The basal ganglia lie deep within the cerebral hemispheres and do not come in contact with the pia mater. Reference *K*, pp. 177 and 178 (Fig. 12:16).

71 Cerebrospinal fluid is manufactured by the:

A. corpus callosum.
B. optic chiasma.
C. internal capsule.
D. choroid plexuses.
E. aqueduct of the midbrain.

72 The plexus from which the ulnar nerve arises is the:

A. brachial.
B. cervical.
C. lumbar.
D. coeliac.
E. choroid.

Answers overleaf

71A

FALSE—The corpus callosum is a tract of nerve fibres which connect the two cerebral hemispheres. Reference *K*, p. 175 (Fig. 12:12).

71B

FALSE—The optic chiasma is where the two optic nerves join within the cranial cavity. Reference *K*, pp. 190 and 191 (Fig. 12:37).

71C

FALSE—The internal capsule is an area of the white matter lying deep within the brain carrying impulses to and from the cerebral cortex. Reference *K*, pp. 175 and 176 (Fig. 12:14).

71D

TRUE—Cerebrospinal fluid is formed by the choroid plexus in each ventricle. Reference *K*, pp. 173 and 174.

71E

FALSE—The aqueduct of the midbrain joins the third ventricle with the fourth ventricle. Reference *K*, p. 173 (Fig. 12:8).

72A

TRUE—The lower four cervical nerves and the majority of the 1st thoracic nerve form the brachial plexus and from this arises the ulnar nerve. Reference *K*, p. 186.

72B

FALSE—The cervical plexus does not provide any of the nerves of the upper limb. Reference *K*, p. 186.

72C

FALSE—The lumbar plexus is concerned with supplying areas of the lower abdomen, thigh and lower limbs. Reference *K*, pp. 187 and 188 (Fig. 12:31).

72D

FALSE—The coeliac plexus supplies sympathetic nerves to a number of viscera and is situated near the coeliac artery. Reference *K*, p. 194 (Fig. 12:40).

72E

FALSE—The choroid plexus is responsible for the manufacture of cerebrospinal fluid. Reference *K*, pp. 173 and 174.

73 The falx cerebri is attached to the:

A. cribriform plate.
B. mastoid process.
C. sphenoid bone.
D. crista galli.
E. clinoid process.

74 The cerebral hemispheres are connected by the corpus:

A. luteum.
B. callosum.
C. albicans.
D. spongiosum.
E. striatum.

Answers overleaf

73A

FALSE—The cribriform plate is the medial part of the horizontal plate of ethmoid and is perforated for the passage of the olfactory nerves. Reference *E*, pp. 34 (Fig. 2.21) and 35.

73B

FALSE—The mastoid process is the lower conical projection of the mastoid part of the temporal bone on the lateral aspect of the skull. Reference *E*, pp. 28 (Fig. 2.15) and 29.

73C

FALSE—The sphenoid bone is situated in the centre of the cranium and lies behind the ethmoid bone. Reference *E*, pp. 32 and 33.

73D

TRUE—The bony projection of the perpendicular plate of ethmoid continued above the horizontal plate is called the crista galli, to which is attached the falx cerebri. Reference *E*, pp. 34 (Fig. 2.21) and 35.

73E

FALSE—The clinoid processes (anterior and posterior) are parts of the sphenoid bone in relation to the hypophyseal fossa. Reference *E*, pp. 32 (Fig. 2.19) and 33.

74A

FALSE—The corpus luteum develops from a Graafian follicle after extrusion of an ovum. Reference *D*, pp. 721 and 722 (Fig. 28–12(a)).

74B

TRUE—The corpus callosum is the internal connection of the two cerebral hemispheres. Reference *D*, pp. 334 (Fig. 14–4) and 336.

74C

FALSE—The corpus albicans is formed from the degenerated corpus luteum in the ovary. Reference *D*, pp. 727 (Fig. 28–17) and 730.

74D

FALSE—The corpus spongiosum is the ventral tissue mass of the penis and contains the spongy urethra. Reference *D*, pp. 718 and 719 (Fig. 28–8).

74E

FALSE—The corpus striatum is the largest of the basal ganglia of the cerebral hemisphere. Reference *D*, pp. 334 (Fig. 14–4) and 339.

75 A conjunction or joining of two adjacent neurons is a:

A. ganglion.
B. synapse.
C. dendrite.
D. plexus.
E. node.

76 The cribriform plate of the ethmoid bone is for the passage of which of the following cranial nerves?

A. 1st.
B. 3rd.
C. 5th.
D. 7th.
E. 9th.

Answers overleaf

75A

FALSE—A ganglion is a group of nerve cell bodies outside the cranial nervous system. Reference *D*, pp. 300 and 303 (Fig. 13–3(a)).

75B

TRUE—The junction between two neurons is called a synapse. Reference *D*, pp. 291 and 292 (Fig. 12–7(c)).

75C

FALSE—A dendrite is a highly branched extension of the cytoplasm of a neurone. Reference *D*, pp. 284 (Fig. 12–2(a)) and 285.

75D

FALSE—A plexus is a network formed from the ventral rami of the spinal nerves. Reference *D*, p. 313 (Fig. 13–11).

75E

FALSE—A node is a swelling caused by a compact mass of tissue, as in a lymph node. Reference *B*, p. 1161.

76A

TRUE—The 1st or olfactory nerve passes through the cribriform plate of ethmoid to the mucosal covering of parts of the nasal cavity. Reference *D*, p. 346.

76B

FALSE—The 3rd or occulomotor nerve passes through the superior orbital fissure of the orbit. Reference *D*, p. 347.

76C

FALSE—The 5th or trigeminal nerve has three branches which pass through the superior orbital fissure, the foramen rotundum and foramen ovale. Reference *D*, p. 347.

76D

FALSE—The 7th or facial nerve passes through the stylomastoid foramen of temporal bone. Reference *D*, p. 157.

76E

FALSE—The 9th or glossopharyngeal nerve passes through the jugular foramen between temporal and occipital bones. Reference *D*, pp. 150 (Fig. 7–4) and 157.

1.8 NEUROLOGY (SPECIAL SENSES)

77 Balance is monitored by the:

A. cerebrum.
B. ossicles.
C. cochlea.
D. semicircular canals.
E. trochlear nerve.

78 In the cerebrum the greater part of the occipital lobe is concerned with the interpretation of:

A. touch.
B. hearing.
C. smell.
D. taste.
E. vision.

Answers overleaf

77A
FALSE—Changes in position of the head are conveyed by nervous impulse to the pons and medulla. Reference *O*, pp. 266 (Table 9–4) and 341.

77B
FALSE—The ossicles in the middle ear are responsible for transmitting sound waves from the tympanic membrane to the fluid within the cochlea. Reference *O*, p. 342.

77C
FALSE—The cochlea is the part of internal ear responsible for hearing. Reference *O*, p. 341.

77D
TRUE—The semicircular canals are concerned with sensing the position of the head and bodily equilibrium. Reference *O*, pp. 341 and 342.

77E
FALSE—The trochlear nerve is the motor nerve for the superior oblique muscle of the eye. Reference *O*, p. 266 (Table 9–4).

78A
FALSE—The interpretation of touch is the responsibility of the cortex of the frontal and parietal lobes adjacent to the central sulcus. Reference *O*, pp. 275 and 279 (Fig. 9–19).

78B
FALSE—The auditory area of the cerebrum is the superior part of the temporal lobe. Reference *O*, p. 279 (Fig. 9–19).

78C
FALSE—The olfactory area is located on the medial aspect of the temporal lobe. Reference *D*, p. 341.

78D
FALSE—The interpretation of taste is the responsibility of the lateral part of the parietal cortex. Reference *D*, p. 341.

78E
TRUE—The interpretation of vision is the responsibility of the occipital lobe. Reference *O*, p. 279 (Fig. 9–19).

79 The auditory (Eustachian) tube connects the:

A. inner ear and pharynx.
B. outer ear and larynx.
C. middle ear and pharynx.
D. inner ear and middle ear.
E. larynx and pharynx.

80 One of the motor nerves that control the eye muscles is the:

A. trochlear.
B. vagus.
C. facial.
D. optic.
E. olfactory.

Answers overleaf

79A
FALSE—The inner ear has no connection to the pharynx. Reference *O*, p. 340.

79B
FALSE—The outer ear has no connection with larynx. Reference *O*, p. 338.

79C
TRUE—The connection between the middle ear and the nasopharynx is the auditory (Eustachian) tube. Reference *O*, pp. 338 (Fig. 11–22) and 340.

79D
FALSE—The middle ear connects with the inner ear via the oval window, into which the stapes fits, and the round window which is covered by a membrane. Reference *O*, p. 339.

79E
FALSE—The laryngopharynx opens directly into the larynx. Reference *O*, pp. 506 and 507 (Fig. 17–7).

80A
TRUE—The trochlear nerve supplies motor fibres to the superior oblique muscle of the eye. Reference *O*, p. 266 (Table 9–4).

80B
FALSE—The motor fibres of the vagus nerve supply the muscles of the pharynx, larynx and thoracic and abdominal viscera. Reference *O*, p. 267 (Table 9–4).

80C
FALSE—The motor fibres of the facial nerve supply the superficial muscles of the face and scalp. Reference *O*, p. 266 (Table 9–4).

80D
FALSE—The optic nerve is the sensory nerve for the retina of the eye. Reference *O*, p. 266 (Table 9–4).

80E
FALSE—The olfactory nerve is sensory and responsible for the sense of smell. Reference *O*, p. 266 (Table 9–4).

81 The cochlea is located within the:

A. parietal bone.
B. sphenoid bone.
C. palatine bone.
D. frontal bone.
E. temporal bone.

82 The middle layer of the eyeball is called the:

A. rectus medialis.
B. choroid.
C. sclera.
D. cornea.
E. retina.

Answers overleaf

81A
FALSE—The parietal bone does not contain any named structures. Reference *O*, pp. 97 and 105.

81B
FALSE—The sphenoid bone only contains the sphenoid sinus. Reference *O*, p. 105.

81C
FALSE—The palatine bones do not contain any named structures. Reference *O*, p. 106.

81D
FALSE—The frontal bone contains the frontal sinuses. Reference *O*, p. 97.

81E
TRUE—The cochlea is located within the petrous portion of the temporal bone. Reference *O*, pp. 105 and 131 (Table 5–3).

82A
FALSE—The rectus medialis is one of the extrinsic muscles of the eye. Reference *O*, pp. 328 and 329 (Fig. 11–11).

82B
TRUE—The choroid is the middle layer of the eyeball containing blood vessels and pigment. Reference *O*, p. 322 and 326 (Table 11–3).

82C
FALSE—The sclera is the outer layer of the eyeball. Reference *O*, pp. 322 and 326 (Table 11–3).

82D
FALSE—The cornea is the transparent anterior part of the sclera. Reference *O*, pp. 322 and 326 (Table 11–3).

82E
FALSE—The retina is the innermost layer of the eyeball. Reference *O*, pp. 324 and 326 (Table 11–3).

83 The point of sharpest vision is found in the:

A. optic disc.
B. centre of the macula lutea.
C. rods of the retina.
D. cones of the retina.
E. choroid.

Answers overleaf

83A

FALSE—The optic disc, in the posterior part of the eyeball, is called the blind spot as light rays striking this area cannot be seen. Reference *O*, pp. 325 and 326.

83B

TRUE—The centre of the macula lutea, the fovea centralis, is the point of sharpest vision. Reference *O*, p. 325.

83C

FALSE—The rods of the retina are responsible for vision in dim light. Reference *O*, p. 336.

83D

FALSE—The cones are responsible for vision in bright light and colour vision, but are less numerous than the rods and are most concentrated in one spot — the fovea centralis. Reference *O*, pp. 325 and 336.

83E

FALSE—The choroid layer is not sensitive to light being a vascular pigmented layer. Reference *O*, p. 326 (Table 11–3).

1.9 RESPIRATORY SYSTEM

84 The air passing in and out of the lungs at quiet breathing is called the:

A. expiratory reserve volume.
B. inspiratory capacity.
C. vital capacity.
D. residual volume.
E. tidal volume.

85 The respiratory centre is *most* sensitive to the:

A. level of haemoglobin in the blood.
B. level of carbon dioxide in the blood.
C. partial pressure of water vapour in inspired air.
D. level of oxygen in the blood.
E. partial pressure of hydrogen in the blood.

Answers overleaf

84A

FALSE—The expiratory reserve volume is the largest additional volume of air that can be forcibly expired after a normal expiration — usually 1000–1200 ml. Reference *O*, pp. 532 and 534 (Fig. 18–9).

84B

FALSE—The inspiratory capacity is the maximum amount of air that can be inspired after a normal expiration — 3500–3800 ml. Reference *O*, p. 535.

84C

FALSE—The vital capacity is the largest volume that can be moved in and out of the lungs — 4500–5000 ml. Reference *O*, p. 534 (Fig. 18–9).

84D

FALSE—The residual volume is that amount of air that cannot be forcibly expired — about 1200 ml. Reference *O*, pp. 532 and 534 (Fig. 18–9).

84E

TRUE—The volume of air exhaled normally after a normal inspiration is called the tidal volume. Reference *O*, pp. 532 and 534 (Fig. 18–9).

85A

FALSE—The level of haemoglobin in the blood determines the amount of oxygen the blood can transport. Reference *O*, p. 539.

85B

TRUE—The chemoreceptors of the respiratory centre located in the medulla respond to small changes in the partial pressure of carbon dioxide to influence respiration. Reference *O*, p. 544.

85C

FALSE—Water vapour pressure plays no part in the control of respiration. Reference *O*, p. 544.

85D

FALSE—The partial pressure of oxygen in the blood does not help regulate respiration under usual conditions, but can help in emergency respiratory control. Reference *O*, p. 544.

85E

FALSE—The pH of blood only affects the oxygen tension by altering the haemoglobin saturation. Reference *O*, p. 541 (Fig. 18–14).

86 The term emphysema refers to:

A. air in the pleural cavity.
B. cavitation of lung tissue.
C. dilatation of the bronchioles.
D. emboli in the pulmonary artery.
E. dilatation of the alveoli.

87 A pneumothorax is:

A. congenital malformation of the pleura.
B. fluid in the pleural cavity.
C. a dust disease of the lung.
D. air in the pleural cavity.
E. blood in the pleural cavity.

Answers overleaf

86A
FALSE—Air in the pleural cavity is termed pneumothorax. Reference *I*, p. 94.

86B
FALSE—Cavitation of lung tissue may be caused by pulmonary tuberculosis or lung abscesses. Reference *I*, pp. 98 and 99.

86C
FALSE—Dilatation of the bronchioles is termed bronchiectasis. Reference *I*, p. 92.

86D
FALSE—Emboli in the pulmonary artery leads to pulmonary embolism. Reference *I*, p. 105.

86E
TRUE—The term emphysema refers to dilatation of the alveoli. Reference *I*, p. 102.

87A
FALSE—Primary disorders of the pleura are uncommon. Reference *I*, p. 93.

87B
FALSE—The presence of fluid in the pleural cavity is termed hydrothorax. Reference *I*, p. 94.

87C
FALSE—The inhalation of dusts produces pneumoconiosis. Reference *I*, pp. 101 and 102.

87D
TRUE—Pneumothorax is a condition where air or other gas is present in the pleural cavity. Reference *I*, p. 94.

87E
FALSE—Bleeding into the pleural cavity is called haemothorax. Reference *I*, p. 94.

1.10 ALIMENTARY SYSTEM

88 Peyer's patches are located in the:

A. stomach.
B. spleen.
C. pancreas.
D. small intestine.
E. kidneys.

89 The primary function of the lacteals is to absorb:

A. amino acids.
B. glucose.
C. fatty acids.
D. sodium chloride.
E. vitamin B.

Answers overleaf

88A
FALSE—The stomach contains gastric glands. Reference *O*, p. 554 (Table 19–1).

88B
FALSE—The spleen is composed of lymphatic tissue and does not contain Peyer's patches. Reference *D*, p. 538.

88C
FALSE—The pancreas contains clusters of endocrine cells called the islets of Langerhans. Reference *O*, p. 584.

88D
TRUE—Clusters of lymph nodes called Peyer's patches are found in the small intestine. Reference *O*, p. 554 (Table 19–1).

88E
FALSE—The kidney contains many named parts of the nephron but not Peyer's patches. Reference *O*, pp. 641 and 642 (Fig. 22–3).

89A
FALSE—Amino acids are absorbed into the blood of the small intestine. Reference *F*, p. 105.

89B
FALSE—Glucose is absorbed into the blood of the small intestine. Reference *F*, p. 105.

89C
TRUE—Fatty acids produced from the fats are primarily absorbed into the intestinal lymphatics called lacteals. Reference *F*, pp. 105 and 106.

89D
FALSE—Sodium chloride is absorbed as the respective ions into the blood stream of the small intestine (90%) and stomach and large intestine (10%). Reference *D*, p. 629.

89E
FALSE—The vitamin B complexes in the diet are all water soluble and absorbed into the blood of the small intestine, or if manufactured by intestinal bacteria, in the large intestine. Reference *D*, pp. 635 and 657.

90 Pancreatic juices enter the duodenum through the:

A. duodenal papilla.
B. islets of Langerhans.
C. pyloric sphincter.
D. ileocaecal valve.
E. cystic duct.

91 Fibrinogen is produced in:

A. the liver.
B. the kidneys.
C. red bone marrow.
D. the spleen.
E. the thymus.

Answers overleaf

90A

TRUE—The pancreatic duct conveys the pancreatic juices into the duodenum via the major duodenal papilla and frequently an accessory minor duodenal papilla. Reference *O*, pp. 583 (Fig. 19–30) and 584.

90B

FALSE—The islets of Langerhans are clusters of exocrine glandular tissue the secretions of which pass into the blood capillaries of the pancreas. Reference *O*, p. 584.

90C

FALSE—The pyloric sphincter guards the opening from the pyloric part of the stomach into the duodenum. Reference *O*, p. 568 (Fig. 19–16).

90D

FALSE—The ileocaecal valve is the opening from the ileum into the caecum. Reference *O*, pp. 574 and 575 (Fig. 19–23).

90E

FALSE—The cystic duct runs from the gall bladder to its junction with the hepatic duct to form the common bile duct, and allows bile to flow into and out of the gall bladder. Reference *O*, pp. 582 and 583 (Fig. 19–30).

91A

TRUE—Fibrinogen, a blood coagulation factor, is produced in the liver. Reference *F*, p. 21.

91B

FALSE—Reference *F*, p. 21.

91C

FALSE—Red bone marrow is one of the sites of production of red blood cells. Reference *F*, p. 9.

91D

FALSE—The spleen is responsible for production of certain blood cells and the destruction of red cells, but not fibrinogen. Reference *F*, p. 157.

91E

FALSE—The thymus is involved in the immunological processes. Reference *F*, pp. 157 and 158.

92 The columns of liver cells in the liver lobule produce:

A. vitamin B_{12}.
B. iron.
C. bile.
D. glycerol.
E. antibodies.

93 Pepsin causes the breakdown of:

A. peptides to amino acids.
B. proteins to polypeptides.
C. polysaccharides to disaccharides.
D. lipids to fatty acids and glycerol.
E. amino acids to ketones.

Answers overleaf

92A
FALSE—Vitamin B_{12} is stored in the liver, but not produced there. Reference *F*, p. 10.

92B
FALSE—Iron can be stored in the liver as ferritin for re-use, but is not produced there. Reference *F*, p. 10.

92C
TRUE—Bile is produced continuously by the liver cells. Reference *F*, p. 109.

92D
FALSE—Glycerol is a component of fat that is obtained during fat metabolism by the liver. Reference *F*, p. 114.

92E
FALSE—Antibodies are produced by the lymphocytes and plasma cells in response to foreign protein. Reference *F*, p. 22.

93A
FALSE—The breakdown of short chain peptides to amino acids is caused by a group of enzymes collectively called erepsin. Reference *F*, p. 105.

93B
TRUE—Food proteins are broken down into polypeptides by the action of pepsin. Reference *F*, p. 105.

93C
FALSE—Polysaccharides are broken down into disaccharides by the action of amylase. Reference *F*, p. 105.

93D
FALSE—Pancreatic lipase is responsible for converting lipids to fatty acids and glycerol. Reference *F*, pp. 105 and 108.

93E
FALSE—Amino acids are deaminated in the liver and elsewhere, not in the digestive tract. Reference *F*, p. 115.

94 Trypsinogen is activated by:

A. lipase.
B. enterokinase.
C. maltase.
D. amylase.
E. peptidase.

95 Vitamin B_{12} absorption depends on:

A. pepsinogen.
B. intrinsic factor.
C. hydrochloric acid.
D. casein.
E. cholecystokinin.

Answers overleaf

94A
FALSE—Lipase is a fat-splitting enzyme found in pancreatic juice with trypsinogen. Reference *F*, p. 108.

94B
TRUE—Trypsinogen is activated by enterokinase, produced by the small intestine, to become trypsin. Reference *F*, p. 108.

94C
FALSE—Maltase, found in pancreatic juice, is responsible for the conversion of maltose to glucose. Reference *F*, pp. 105 and 108.

94D
FALSE—Amylase, found in pancreatic juice, acts on starch to produce disaccharides. Reference *F*, pp. 105 and 108.

94E
FALSE—Peptidases are inactive forms of enzymes secreted by the intestinal cells which require activation themselves. Reference *O*, pp. 595, 596 and 597 (Fig. 20–2).

95A
FALSE—Pepsinogen is the inactive form of pepsin, a proteolytic enzyme. Reference *O*, p. 595 (Table 20–2).

95B
TRUE—Intrinsic factor, produced by the gastric mucosa, is necessary for the absorption of Vitamin B_{12}. Reference *O*, pp. 400, 570 and 592.

95C
FALSE—Hydrochloric acid provides the acid environment in the stomach for enzyme activation. Reference *O*, p. 595 (Table 20–2).

95D
FALSE—Casein is a protein derived from milk. Reference *O*, pp. 595 (Table 20–2) and *F*, p. 106.

95E
FALSE—Cholecystokinin is a humoral agent released when fat enters the duodenum and causes the gall bladder to contract. Reference *F*, p. 109.

96 Lipase acts on:

A. sugar.
B. protein.
C. starch.
D. carbohydrates.
E. fat.

97 Rickets is a disease which is due to the lack of:

A. vitamin A.
B. vitamin B_{12}.
C. vitamin C.
D. vitamin D.
E. vitamin E.

Answers overleaf

96A

FALSE—Sugar (sucrose) is acted upon by sucrase and converted to glucose and fructose. Reference *F*, p. 105.

96B

FALSE—Protein requires proteases to commence the breakdown. Reference *O*, p. 595 (Table 20–2).

96C

FALSE—Starch is acted upon by amylase, found in saliva and pancreatic juice. Reference *O*, p. 595 (Table 20–2).

96D

FALSE—Lipase does not act on carbohydrates. Reference *O*, pp. 595 (Table 20–2) and 596.

96E

TRUE—Lipase, found in gastric and pancreatic juices, acts on fat to produce fatty acids and glycerol. Reference *O*, p. 595 (Table 20–2).

97A

FALSE—Vitamin A deficiency leads to epithelial disorders, night blindness or faulty bone and teeth development. Reference *D*, p. 656.

97B

FALSE—Vitamin B_{12} deficiency leads to pernicious anaemia and nervous system malfunction. Reference *D*, p. 657.

97C

FALSE—Vitamin C deficiency leads to scurvy. Reference *D*, p. 657.

97D

TRUE—Vitamin D deficiency in children leads to rickets (defective utilisation of calcium by bone). Termed osteomalacia in adults. Reference *D*, p. 656.

97E

FALSE—Vitamin E deficiency leads to haemolytic anaemia. Reference *D*, p. 656.

1.11 URINARY SYSTEM

98 Renal lithiasis means:

A. inflammation of kidney tissue.
B. a calculus in the kidney.
C. carcinoma of the renal cortex.
D. pus in the renal pelvis.
E. retention of urine.

99 The term enuresis means:

A. excess formation of urine.
B. difficulty in micturition.
C. blood in the urine.
D. involuntary passage of urine.
E. painful micturition.

Answers overleaf

98A
FALSE—Inflammation of the renal substance is termed nephritis. Reference *I*, pp. 154 and 156.

98B
TRUE—Renal lithiasis means a calculus in the kidney. Reference *I*, p. 159.

98C
FALSE—Adenocarcinoma is a carcinomatous growth of the solid part of the kidney in adult life. Reference *I*, p. 157.

98D
FALSE—Pus in the renal pelvis is termed pyonephrosis. Reference *I*, p. 155.

98E
FALSE—Retention of urine is a clinical sign and a symptom of an obstructive condition. Reference *I*, pp. 150, 159 and 160.

99A
FALSE—Formation of greater than normal amounts of urine is diuresis. Reference *I*, p. 216.

99B
FALSE—Difficulty in passing urine is dysuria. Reference *I*, p. 150.

99C
FALSE—Blood in the urine is haematuria. Reference *I*, p. 150.

99D
TRUE—The involuntary voiding of urine is enuresis. Reference *B*, p. 598.

99E
FALSE—Painful micturition is called dysuria. Reference *B*, p. 557.

100 An 'ectopic' kidney refers to:

A. a non-functioning kidney.
B. a kidney abnormally placed.
C. an abnormally small kidney.
D. one kidney with two ureters.
E. the two kidneys joined together.

101 The serous coat of the urinary bladder is:

A. continuous with the mucous membrane lining the ureters and urethra.
B. constructed of three layers of muscle fibres.
C. a partial one and derived from peritoneum.
D. a layer of loose areolar tissue connecting the other coats.
E. composed of transitional epithelium.

Answers overleaf

100A
FALSE—Reference *I*, p. 153.

100B
TRUE—An abnormally placed kidney in the lower abdomen or pelvic cavity is called an ectopic kidney. Reference *I*, p. 153.

100C
FALSE—A kidney which fails to develop normally in size is called a congenital hypoplastic kidney. Reference *I*, p. 153.

100D
FALSE—A kidney with two ureters would result as part of the anomaly called duplex kidney. Reference *I*, p. 153.

100E
FALSE—Partial fusion between the lower poles of the two kidneys is called horseshoe kidney. Reference *I*, p. 153.

101A
FALSE—The mucous membrane is an internal lining, the serous coat of the bladder is external. Reference *O*, pp. 660–662.

101B
FALSE—Three layers of muscle fibres constitute the bladder wall Reference *O*, p. 661.

101C
TRUE—The serous membrane forming the parietal peritoneum covers only the superior surface of the bladder. Reference *O*, p. 661.

101D
FALSE—The serous coat is epithelial in origin whilst areolar tissue is connective. Reference *O*, p. 68 (Table 3–1).

101E
FALSE—Transitional epithelium is the surface of the mucous membrane lining the urinary bladder. Reference *O*, p. 68 (Table 3–1).

102 The term 'cystitis' means inflammation of the:

A. cystic duct.
B. gall bladder.
C. urinary bladder.
D. basal cistern.
E. renal pelvis.

103 Transitional cell carcinoma occurs in which of the following?

A. Uterine (fallopian) tubes.
B. Bladder.
C. Rectum.
D. Ovary.
E. Urethra.

Answers overleaf

102A
FALSE—Inflammation of the cystic and other bile ducts is known as cholangitis. Reference *I*, p. 142.

102B
FALSE—Inflammation of the gall bladder is known as cholecystitis. Reference *I*, p. 140.

102C
TRUE—Cystitis means inflammation of the urinary bladder. Reference *I*, p. 165.

102D
FALSE—Inflammation of the basal cistern would be termed meningitis. Reference *I*, pp. 53 and 277.

102E
FALSE—Inflammation of the renal pelvis is termed pyelitis. Reference *I*, p. 154.

103A
FALSE—The uterine tubes have a lining of ciliated columnar epithelium and carcinoma of the uterine tubes is uncommon. Reference *O*, pp. 737, 738 and 739 (Fig. 27–7) and *I*, p. 182.

103B
TRUE—A carcinomatous growth of the epithelial lining of the bladder is a transitional cell carcinoma. Reference *I*, p. 166.

103C
FALSE—The rectal lining is simple columnar epithelium and carcinoma of the large intestine occurs in the rectum. Reference *I*, p. 130.

103D
FALSE—Transitional cell carcinoma is not found in the ovary. Reference *I*, p. 180.

103E
FALSE—Carcinoma of the urethra is very rare. Reference *I*, p. 169.

1.12 REPRODUCTIVE SYSTEM

104 Salpingitis is inflammation of the:

A. uterine (fallopian) tubes.
B. uterus.
C. vagina.
D. cervix.
E. ovary.

105 A function of the prostate gland is to:

A. support the urinary bladder.
B. produce a thin lubricant fluid.
C. excrete urine.
D. produce hormonal secretions.
E. store sperm.

Answers overleaf

104A
TRUE—Inflammation of the uterine tubes is termed salpingitis. Reference *I*, p. 178.

104B
FALSE—Endometritis is the term to describe inflammation of the uterus. Reference *I*, p. 179.

104C
FALSE—Vaginitis is inflammation of the vagina. Reference *I*, p.179.

104D
FALSE—Cervicitis is the term to denote inflammation of the cervix. Reference *I*, p. 179.

104E
FALSE—Inflammation of the ovaries, frequently accompanied by inflammation of the uterine tubes is more correctly called salpingo-oophoritis. Reference *I*, p. 178.

105A
FALSE—The urinary bladder is a freely movable organ held in position by the folds of peritoneum. Reference *D*, p. 689.

105B
TRUE—The prostate gland is responsible for producing a thin alkaline fluid for protection of sperm and lubrication. Reference *D*, p. 718.

105C
FALSE—The nephrons of the kidney are responsible for the urine excretion. Reference *D*, p. 676.

105D
FALSE—The prostate gland is not classified as a ductless gland and does not open directly into the blood. Reference *D*, pp. 718 and 719 (Fig. 28–8).

105E
FALSE—The epididymis is responsible for sperm maturation and storage. Reference *D*, p. 715.

106 Fibroids are found in the:

A. ovary.
B. rectum.
C. vagina.
D. peritoneal cavity.
E. uterus.

107 The internal os of the uterus marks the junction of:

A. uterine tube and peritoneal cavity.
B. uterine tube and fundus of uterus.
C. fundus and body of uterus.
D. body and cervix of uterus.
E. cervix and vagina.

Answers overleaf

106A
FALSE—There are many primary ovarian neoplasms, but none are referred to as fibroids. Reference *I*, p. 180.

106B
FALSE—Benign neoplasm of the rectum is termed a polyp. Reference *I*, p. 129.

106C
FALSE—Benign tumours of the vagina are rare. Reference *Q*, p. 422.

106D
FALSE—Primary tumours of the peritoneum are exceedingly rare. Reference *Q*, p. 221.

106E
TRUE—Benign tumours of the uterus are referred to as fibroids. Reference *I*, p. 180.

107A
FALSE—The part of the uterine tube that opens into the peritoneal cavity is called the infundibulum. Reference *O*, p. 737.

107B
FALSE—The part of the uterine tube that meets the uterus just below the fundus is called the isthmus. Reference *O*, p. 737.

107C
FALSE—The fundus is the upper part of the body above the uterine tubes. Reference *O*, p. 734.

107D
TRUE—The internal os of the uterus is the junction of the uterine cavity and the cervical canal. Reference *O*, p. 734.

107E
FALSE—The external os is the constricted lower end of the cervix where it opens into the vagina. Reference *O*, p. 734.

108 Convoluted seminiferous tubules are found in the:

A. prostate gland.
B. epididymis.
C. spermatic cord.
D. seminal vesicles.
E. testis.

109 Ducts from the prostate gland open into the:

A. urethra.
B. seminal vesicles.
C. testes.
D. scrotum.
E. epididymis.

Answers overleaf

108A
FALSE—The prostate is a compound tubuloalveolar gland. Reference *O*, pp. 65 (Fig. 3–6) and 726.

108B
FALSE—The epididymis is a single coiled tube. Reference *O*, pp. 722 and 723 (Fig. 26–7).

108C
FALSE—The spermatic cord is a cylindrical casing of white fibrous tissue enclosing the vas deferens, blood vessels, lymphatics and nerves. Reference *O*, p. 727.

108D
FALSE—The seminal vesicles are convoluted pouches lying posterior to the bladder and in front of the rectum. Reference *O*, pp. 718 (Fig. 26–2) and 726.

108E
TRUE—Convoluted seminiferous tubules are found in the lobules of the testis. Reference *O*, pp. 717 and 718 (Fig. 26–1).

109A
TRUE—The ducts from the prostate gland open into the prostatic urethra. Reference *D*, p. 718.

109B
FALSE—The seminal vesicles open into the ejaculatory duct. Reference *D*, p. 718.

109C
FALSE—The testes are in the scrotum, outside the body, whilst the prostate gland is an internal gland. Reference *D*, p. 710 (Fig. 28–1).

109D
FALSE—The scrotum is a pouch of the abdominal wall containing the testis, epididymis and ductus (vas) deferens. Reference *D*, p. 710

109E
FALSE—The epididymis lies between the testis and the ductus (vas) deferens in the scrotum. Reference *D*, p. 711 (Fig. 28–2(a)).

1.13 ENDOCRINE SYSTEM

110 The gland secreting the antidiuretic hormone is the:

A. suprarenal cortex.
B. parathyroid.
C. thyroid.
D. thymus.
E. posterior lobe of pituitary.

111 Which of the following glands uses iodine in the manufacture of a hormone?

A. Anterior lobe of pituitary.
B. Posterior lobe of pituitary.
C. Parathyroid.
D. Suprarenal.
E. Thyroid.

Answers overleaf

110A
FALSE—The suprarenal cortex secretes mineralocorticoids, glucocorticoids and gonadocorticoids. Reference *O*, p. 374.

110B
FALSE—The parathyroid secretes parathyroid hormone. Reference *O*, p. 373.

110C
FALSE—The thyroid secretes thyroid hormones and calcitonin. Reference *O*, pp. 370 and 371.

110D
FALSE—The thymus secretes thymosin. Reference *O*, p. 382.

110E
TRUE—The posterior lobe of pituitary (neurohypophysis) is responsible for the secretion of the antidiuretic hormone into the blood stream. Reference *O*, p. 364.

111A
FALSE—The hormones of the anterior lobe of the pituitary gland are all proteins or polypeptides and do not contain minerals. Reference *R*, p. 27.12.

111B
FALSE—The hormones of the posterior lobe of the pituitary gland are polypeptides and do not contain minerals. Reference *R*, p. 27.16.

111C
FALSE—Parathyroid hormone is a polypeptide without inorganic minerals. Reference *R*, p. 27.26.

111D
FALSE—The hormones of the suprarenal cortex are steroids and those of the medulla are amine derivatives — all organic. Reference *R*, p. 27.1.

111E
TRUE—The thyroid gland manufactures thyroxine and triiodothyronine produced from an amino acid and inorganic iodine. Reference *R*, p. 27.17.

112 The posterior lobe of the pituitary gland releases:

A. follicle stimulating hormone.
B. prolactin (lactogenic hormone).
C. thyroid stimulating hormone.
D. oxytocin.
E. luteinising hormone.

Answers overleaf

112A

FALSE— Follicle stimulating hormone is secreted by the anterior lobe of the pituitary gland. Reference *O*, p. 357 (Fig. 12–4).

112B

FALSE—Prolactin is secreted by the anterior lobe of the pituitary gland. Reference *O*, p. 357 (Fig. 12–4).

112C

FALSE—Thyroid stimulating hormone is secreted by the anterior lobe of the pituitary gland. Reference *O*, p. 357 (Fig. 12–4).

112D

TRUE—The posterior lobe of the pituitary gland releases oxytocin. Reference *O*, pp. 366 and 368 (Table 12–2).

112E

FALSE—Luteinising hormone is secreted by the anterior lobe of the pituitary gland. Reference *O*, p. 357 (Fig. 12–4).

1.14 SURFACE MARKINGS AND LEVELS

113 The apex beat of the heart is normally to the left of the midline at the level of the:

A. 4th rib.
B. 4th intercostal space.
C. 5th rib.
D. 5th intercostal space.
E. 6th rib.

114 The hilum of the left kidney lies at the level of:

A. 10th thoracic vertebra (TV 10).
B. TV 12.
C. 1st lumbar vertebra (LV 1).
D. LV 3.
E. LV 5.

Answers overleaf

113A
FALSE—Reference *S*, p. 58.

113B
FALSE—Reference *S*, p. 58.

113C
FALSE—Reference *S*, p. 58.

113D
TRUE—The apex beat of the heart is 9 cm to the left of the midline in the 5th intercostal space. Reference *S*, p. 58.

113E
FALSE—Reference *S*, p. 58.

114A
FALSE—At the level of 10th thoracic vertebra is the oesophageal opening of the diaphragm. Reference *S*, p. 72.

114B
FALSE—The level of 12th thoracic vertebra is the point of origin of the coeliac artery on the anterior aspect of the aorta. Reference *S*, p. 82.

114C
TRUE—The hilum of the left kidney lies at the level of 1st lumbar vertebra. Reference *S*, p. 80 (Fig. 42).

114D
FALSE—The level of 3rd lumbar vertebra is the lower pole of the kidneys. Reference *S*, p. 80 (Fig. 42).

114E
FALSE—The level of 5th lumbar vertebra is the level of the ileocaecal valve, where the transtubercular and right lateral planes intersect. Reference *S*, pp. 77 and 104.

115 In the extended knee, the relationship of the tibial tubercle to the apex of the patella is:

A. 1 cm below.
B. 1 cm laterally.
C. immediately below.
D. 5 cm below.
E. 5 cm laterally.

116 The transpyloric plane lies at the level of the lower border of:

A. 1st lumbar vertebra (LV 1).
B. LV 2.
C. LV 3.
D. LV 4.
E. LV 5.

Answers overleaf

115A
FALSE—Reference *T*, p. 348.

115B
FALSE—Reference *T*, p. 348.

115C
FALSE—Reference *T*, p. 348.

115D
TRUE—The tibial tubercle is 5 cm below the apex of the patella in the extended knee. Reference *T*, p. 348.

115E
FALSE—Reference *T*, p. 348.

116A
TRUE—The transpyloric plane approximates to the lower border of 1st lumbar vertebra. Reference *S*, pp. 67 and 78 (Fig. 39).

116B
FALSE—The lower border of 2nd lumbar vertebra lies at the level of the subcostal plane. Reference *S*, pp. 67 and 78 (Fig. 39).

116C
FALSE—The lower border of 3rd lumbar vertebra approximates to the lower pole of the right kidney. Reference *S*, pp. 79 and 80 (Fig. 42).

116D
FALSE—The lower border of 4th lumbar vertebra approximates to the level of the subcristal plane. Reference *S*, p. 67.

116E
FALSE—The lower border of 5th lumbar vertebra approximates to the level of the transtubercular plane. Reference *S*, pp. 67 and 68 (Fig. 30).

117 The cricoid cartilage lies at the vertebral level of:

A. 2nd cervical.
B. 4th cervical.
C. 5th cervical.
D. 6th cervical.
E. 1st thoracic.

Answers overleaf

117A
FALSE—This is too high a level for the cricoid cartilage. Reference *S*, p. 50.

117B
FALSE—This level is for the upper border of the thyroid cartilage. Reference *S*, p. 50.

117C
FALSE—Reference *S*, p. 50.

117D
TRUE—The cricoid cartilage lies at the level of 6th cervical vertebra. Reference *S*, p. 50.

117E
FALSE—The 1st thoracic vertebra is taken as the posterior level of the superior thoracic aperture. Reference *S*, p. 56.

1.15 REGIONS AND RELATIONS

118 The epigastric region of the body lies between the:

A. right and left lumbar regions.
B. right and left iliac regions.
C. right and left hypochondriac regions.
D. umbilical and hypogastric regions.
E. umbilical and right iliac regions.

119 The hilum of the left kidney is related to the:

A. splenic flexure of the colon.
B. stomach.
C. spleen.
D. pancreas.
E. jejunum.

Answers overleaf

118A

FALSE—The umbilical region lies between the right and left lumbar regions. Reference *T*, p. 68 (Fig. 30).

118B

FALSE—The hypogastric region lies between the right and left iliac regions. Reference *T*, p. 68 (Fig. 30).

118C

TRUE—The epigastric region lies between the right and left hypochondriac regions. Reference *T*, p. 68 (Fig. 30).

118D

FALSE—The transtubercular plane separates the umbilical and hypogastric regions. Reference *T*, p. 68 (Fig. 30).

118E

FALSE—The right iliac region is diagonally below the umbilical region. Reference *T*, p. 68 (Fig. 30).

119A

FALSE—The splenic flexure of the colon lies beneath the lower end of the spleen on the left side of the abdomen. Reference *D*, pp. 17 (Fig. 1–5(c)), 622 (Fig. 24–15) and 633.

119B

FALSE—The pancreas lies between the stomach anteriorly and the kidney posteriorly. Reference *D*, p. 18 (Fig. 1–5(d)).

119C

FALSE—The spleen lies superiorly and laterally to the hilum of the left kidney. Reference *D*, pp. 18 (Fig. 1–5(d)) and 622 (Fig. 24–15).

119D

TRUE—The pancreas is related to the hilum of the left kidney. Reference *D*, p. 622 (Fig. 24–15).

119E

FALSE—The jejunum lies below the transverse colon and anteriorly in the abdominal cavity. Reference *D*, pp. 16 (Fig. 1–5(b)) and 17 (Fig. 1–5(d)).

120 The caecum is:

A. in the left iliac region.
B. in the right hypochondrium.
C. a midline structure in the abdomen.
D. in the right iliac region.
E. attached to the jejunum.

121 The thymus lies immediately posterior to the:

A. sternum.
B. heart.
C. aortic arch.
D. trachea.
E. thyroid gland.

Answers overleaf

120A
FALSE—The left iliac region contains parts of the descending and sigmoid colon and small intestine. Reference *D*, p. 16 (Fig. 1–5(b)).

120B
FALSE—The right hypochondriac region contains part of the right lobe of the liver, the gall bladder and the upper part of the right kidney. Reference *D*, p. 16 (Fig. 1–5(b)).

120C
FALSE—The caecum lies on the right side of the abdomen. Reference *D*, p. 17 (Fig. 1–5(c)).

120D
TRUE—The right iliac region contains the lower part of the caecum. Reference *D*, p. 17 (Fig. 1–5(c)).

120E
FALSE—The jejunum lies in the umbilical region and is a continuation of the duodenum and becomes the ileum. It is not attached to the caecum. Reference *D*, pp. 17 and 620.

121A
TRUE—The thymus is located in the superior and anterior mediastinum and is posterior to the sternum. Reference *D*, pp. 15 (Fig. 1–4(a)) and 429.

121B
FALSE—The thymus is in front of and above the heart. Posterior to the heart is the posterior mediastinum. Reference *D*, pp. 15 (Fig. 1–4(a)) and 429 (Fig. 18–20).

121C
FALSE—The arch of the aorta lies in the superior mediastinum and is posterior to the thymus. Reference *D*, p. 15 (Fig. 1–4(a)).

121D
FALSE—The trachea lies in the posterior mediastinum and the thymus is anterior in relationship. Reference *D*, p. 15 (Fig. 1–4(a)).

121E
FALSE—The thyroid gland is located anteriorly in the neck and outside the mediastinum. It is superior in relationship to the thymus. Reference *D*, p. 419 (Fig. 18–7).

122 The gall bladder lies partly on the:

A. inferior surface of the left lobe of the liver.
B. inferior surface of the right dome of the diaphragm.
C. anterior surface of the left kidney.
D. inferior surface of the right lobe of the liver.
E. superior surface of the pancreas.

123 In anterior relation to the pancreas is the:

A. aorta.
B. left kidney.
C. left suprarenal gland.
D. stomach.
E. inferior vena cava.

Answers overleaf

122A
FALSE—The gall bladder lies on the right side of the body. Reference *D*, p. 617 (Fig. 24–13(a)).

122B
FALSE—The inferior surface of the right dome of the diaphragm is in contact with the upper surface of the right lobe of the liver. Reference *D*, pp. 616 and 617 (Fig. 24–13(a)).

122C
FALSE—The gall bladder is a right-sided organ. Reference *D*, p. 17 (Fig. 1–5(c)).

122D
TRUE—The gall bladder lies partly on the inferior surface of the right lobe of the liver. Reference *D*, pp. 17 (Fig. 1–5(c)) and 617 (Fig. 24–13(a)).

122E
FALSE—The gall bladder is separated from the head of pancreas by the duodenum. The gall bladder lies to the right and the pancreas lies centrally and to the left in the abdomen. Reference *D*, pp. 16, 17 (Fig. 1–5(c)) and 18 (Fig. 1–5(d)).

123A
FALSE—The abdominal aorta is posterior to the pancreas. Reference *D*, p. 622 (Fig. 24–15).

123B
FALSE—The left kidney is posterior to the pancreas. Reference *D*, pp. 18 (Fig. 1–5(d)) and 622 (Fig. 24–15).

123C
FALSE—The left suprarenal gland is posterior to the tail of the pancreas. Reference *D*, p. 18 (Fig. 1–5(d)).

123D
TRUE—The greater curvature of the stomach lies anterior to the pancreas. Reference *D*, pp. 18 (Fig. 1–5(d)) and 615.

123E
FALSE—The inferior vena cava lies posterior to the head of pancreas. Reference *D*, pp. 18 (Fig. 1–5(d)) and 622 (Fig. 24–15).

SECTION 2

Introduction

Each question consists of a stem, followed by 3 options. ONE, TWO or ALL THREE options may be correct for the particular stem.

In this section, the option is denoted by the term TRUE, if it is correct, and by the term FALSE if it is not correct.

In the examination, candidates are required to mark their selection in ONE of 5 boxes labelled **A** to **E** inclusive.

Remember ALL options must be considered to determine whether they are true or false BEFORE making the selection for the examination.

The instruction that introduces this type of question in the examination is as follows:

For each of the following questions or incomplete statements, ONE or MORE of the responses given are correct.

Decide which of the responses is/are correct.

Then choose:

A if all are correct.
B if only numbers 1 and 2 are correct.
C if only numbers 2 and 3 are correct.
D if only number 1 is correct.
E if only number 3 is correct.

2.1 CYTOLOGY

124 Which of the following is a/are serous membrane(s)?

1. Peritoneum.
2. Pleura.
3. Pericardium.

125 Factors essential for the coagulation of blood include:

1. vitamin D.
2. calcium ions.
3. prothrombin.

126 The skin:

1. forms a protective covering for the body.
2. plays a part in the regulation of body temperature.
3. secretes sebum.

Answers overleaf

124.1
TRUE—The peritoneum is a large, continuous sheet of serous membrane, lining the walls of the abdominal cavity and the outer coat of the organs. Reference *O*, p. 574.

124.2
TRUE—The pleura consists of parietal and visceral layers of serous membrane in the thoracic cavity. Reference *O*, p. 519.

124.3
TRUE—The pericardium has a fibrous and serous portion. The serous portion has parietal and visceral layers between which is a potential pericardial space. Reference *O*, p. 421.

125.1
FALSE—Vitamin D is essential for the absorption and utilisation of calcium and phosphorus from the digestive tract. Reference *D*, p. 656.

125.2
TRUE—Calcium ions are an essential factor for the conversion of prothrombin to thrombin. Reference *O*, p. 409.

125.3
TRUE— Prothrombin, produced by the liver, is essential for conversion to the plasma enzyme thrombin in blood coagulation. Reference *O*, p. 409.

126.1
TRUE—One function of the skin is to form a protective covering for the body. Reference *D*, p. 106.

126.2
TRUE—The skin helps to control body temperature. Reference *D*, pp. 113 and 114.

126.3
TRUE—The sebaceous glands, connected to hair follicles, secrete sebum. Reference *D*, p. 112.

127 Examples of connective tissue are:

1. blood.
2. bone.
3. adipose tissue.

128 Pathogenic micro-organisms include:

1. bacteria.
2. fungi.
3. viruses.

129 Metastases may spread via the:

1. lymph.
2. cerebrospinal fluid.
3. blood.

Answers overleaf

127.1
TRUE—Blood is classified as a type of connective tissue. Reference *O*, p. 69.

127.2
TRUE—Bone is a type of connective tissue giving support and protection. Reference *O*, p. 68.

127.3
TRUE—Adipose tissue is a connective tissue that protects, insulates and acts as a storage depot for excess food. Reference *O*, pp. 68 and 70.

128.1
TRUE—Bacteria are one of the main varieties of pathogens. Reference *I*, p. 33.

128.2
TRUE—Some fungi are classified as pathogenic micro-organisms, e.g. ringworm, athlete's foot. Reference *I*, p. 34.

128.3
TRUE—Viruses are an example of a pathogenic micro-organism. Reference *I*, p. 34.

129.1
TRUE—Metastatic spread may occur via the lymph and lymphatics. Reference *I*, p. 41.

129.2
TRUE—The cerebrospinal fluid is a route of spread of tumours of the nervous system. Reference *Q*, p. 626.

129.3
TRUE—The blood in the bloodstream is one route of metastatic spread. Reference *I*, p. 41.

130 Transitional epithelium is found lining the:

1. pelvis of the kidney.
2. urinary bladder.
3. epidermis of the skin.

131 Bone marrow produces:

1. erythrocytes.
2. leucocytes.
3. thrombocytes.

Answers overleaf

130.1
TRUE—The pelvis of the kidney, apart from the renal papillae, has a lining of transitional epithelium. Reference *R*, pp. 35.12 (Plate 35.1(b)) and 36.3.

130.2
TRUE—The inner coat, the mucosa, of the urinary bladder is transitional epithelium, to allow stretching of the wall. Reference *D*, p. 689.

130.3
FALSE—The epidermis of the skin is composed of stratified squamous epithelium, to offer protection. Reference *D*, p. 107.

131.1
TRUE—Red bone marrow in the adult is responsible for producing red blood cells (erythrocytes). Reference *D*, p. 443.

131.2
TRUE—Leucocytes, both granular and agranular, are produced within the red bone marrow. Reference *D*, p. 443.

131.3
TRUE—Thrombocytes (platelets) are produced by red bone marrow. Reference *D*, p. 443.

2.2 OSTEOLOGY

132 The roof of the nasal cavity is formed by the:

1. vomer.
2. sphenoid.
3. ethmoid.

133 The first cervical vertebra has a:

1. foramen transversarium.
2. posterior and anterior arch.
3. heart-shaped body.

134 The sacrum in the adult:

1. contains the spinal cord in the sacral canal.
2. is formed by the fusion of five sacral vertebrae.
3. forms part of the true pelvis.

135 Features of the clavicle include:

1. ossification in membrane.
2. absence of a medullary cavity.
3. articulation with the scapular coracoid process.

Answers overleaf

132.1
FALSE—The vomer, a roughly triangular bone, forms the inferior and posterior part of the nasal septum. Reference *D*, pp. 154 (Fig. 7–7(a)) and 156.

132.2
TRUE—The anterior part of the body of the sphenoid forms the posterior part of the roof of the nasal cavity. Reference *D*, pp. 154 (Fig. 7–7(a)) and 556 (Fig. 23–2(b)).

132.3
TRUE—The cribriform plate of ethmoid forms part of the roof of the nasal cavity. Reference *D*, pp. 152 (Fig. 7–6(a)) and 153.

133.1
TRUE—The transverse processes of the first cervical vertebra are pierced by the transverse foramina. Reference *D*, pp. 162 (Fig. 7–13(b)) and 163.

133.2
TRUE—The first cervical vertebra possesses an anterior and posterior arch. Reference *D*, pp. 162 (Fig. 7–13(b)) and 163.

133.3
FALSE—The first cervical vertebra does not have a body. Reference *D*, p. 163.

134.1
FALSE—The spinal cord ends at the level of the 2nd lumbar vertebra, and the sacral canal contains the sacral nerves. Reference *D*, pp. 300 and 301 (Fig. 13–1).

134.2
TRUE—The sacrum is formed by the fusion of five sacral vertebrae. Reference *D*, pp. 165 and 166 (Fig. 7–16).

134.3
TRUE—The sacrum forms the posterior portion of the true pelvis. Reference *D*, p. 183.

135.1
TRUE—The clavicle is a long bone but is ossified from membrane. Reference *G*, p. 44.

135.2
TRUE—The clavicle has no medullary cavity. Reference *G*, p. 44.

135.3
FALSE—The lateral extremity articulates with the acromion process of scapula to form the acromioclavicular joint. Reference *G*, p. 45.

136 The sphenoid bone contains the foramen:

1. magnum.
2. spinosum.
3. rotundum.

137 Typical cervical vertebrae have:

1. a vertebral canal smaller than that of the thoracic vertebrae.
2. a bifid spinous process.
3. an oval rather than a round body.

138 In the female pelvis the:

1. bones are lighter and smaller than in the male.
2. subpubic angle is greater than in the male.
3. pelvic cavity is deep and funnel-shaped.

Answers overleaf

136.1
FALSE—The foramen magnum is found in the occipital bone. Reference *G*, p. 146.

136.2
TRUE—The foramen spinosum is found in the greater wing of sphenoid and transmits the meningeal artery and nerve. Reference *G*, p. 148.

136.3
TRUE—The foramen rotundum on the greater wing of sphenoid is for the maxillary nerve. Reference *G*, p. 148.

137.1
FALSE—The vertebral canal is large and triangular to accommodate the cervical enlargement of the spinal cord, and is larger than the thoracic vertebrae. Reference *G*, pp. 106 and 110.

137.2
TRUE—The spinous process of a typical cervical vertebra is bifid (divided). Reference *G*, p. 106.

137.3
TRUE—The body of a typical cervical vertebra is oval in shape. Reference *G*, p. 106.

138.1
TRUE—The bones of the female pelvis are lighter and smaller than in the male. Reference *E*, p. 211.

138.2
TRUE—The subpubic angle (the angle below the symphysis between the inferior rami of the pubic bones) is greater than in the male. Reference *E*, p. 211.

138.3
FALSE—The pelvic cavity in the female is short and cylindrical. Reference *G*, p. 86 (Table 7.1).

2.3 ARTHROLOGY

139 Movements at the elbow joint include:

1. flexion.
2. circumduction.
3. abduction.

140 Synovial pivot joints allow:

1. rotation.
2. flexion.
3. extension.

141 Typical features of a synovial joint are:

1. a fibrous capsule.
2. hyaline cartilage.
3. synovial fluid.

142 Articulating surfaces in the knee joint are the:

1. posterior aspect of the patella.
2. distal end of the femur.
3. proximal end of fibula.

Answers overleaf

139.1
TRUE—The elbow joint, being a synovial hinge joint, is capable of flexion. Reference *G*, p. 38.

139.2
FALSE—Circumduction, a circular movement involving a combination of flexion, extension, abduction and adduction, is not possible at the elbow joint. Reference *E*, pp. 2 and 164.

139.3
FALSE—Abduction, a movement away from the midline of the body, is not possible at the elbow joint. Reference *E*, pp. 2 and 164.

140.1
TRUE—Rotation is a movement possible in a synovial pivot joint. Reference *G*, p. 12.

140.2
FALSE—Flexion is not possible in a pivot joint, the only movement is rotation. Reference *G*, p. 12.

140.3
FALSE—Extension is not possible in a pivot joint, the only movement is rotation. Reference *G*, p. 12.

141.1
TRUE—A fibrous capsule surrounds a synovial joint. Reference *G*, pp. 10 (Fig. 2.1) and 11.

141.2
TRUE—Hyaline cartilage covers the articular surfaces of a synovial joint. Reference *G*, pp. 10 (Fig. 2.1) and 11.

141.3
TRUE—Synovial fluid, a lubricant, is secreted by the synovial membrane. Reference *G*, pp. 10 (Fig. 2.1) and 11.

142.1
TRUE—The posterior aspect of the patella is an articulating surface in the knee joint. Reference *G*, p. 70.

142.2
TRUE—The medial and lateral condyles on the distal end of the femur are articulating surfaces in the knee joint. Reference *G*, p. 70.

142.3
FALSE—The proximal end of the fibula forms part of the superior tibiofibular joint. Reference *G*, p. 76.

2.4 MYOLOGY

143 Extension of the elbow joint is produced by the:

1. brachialis muscle.
2. coracobrachialis muscle.
3. triceps muscle.

144 Muscles involved in inspiration include the:

1. diaphragm.
2. scalene muscle.
3. external intercostal muscles.

145 In addition to the aorta, the aortic opening of the diaphragm transmits the:

1. inferior vena cava.
2. oesophagus.
3. thoracic duct.

146 Features of voluntary muscle include:

1. spindle-shaped cells.
2. a covering of sarcolemma.
3. more than one nucleus.

Answers overleaf

143.1
FALSE—The brachialis muscle is a flexor of the elbow joint. Reference *E*, p. 164.

143.2
FALSE—The coracobrachialis muscle is a flexor and adductor of the arm. Reference *E*, p. 142.

143.3
TRUE—The triceps muscle is responsible for extension of the elbow joint in association with the anconeus. Reference *E*, pp. 164 and 165.

144.1
TRUE—The diaphragm is the major muscle of inspiration. Reference *E*, p. 129.

144.2
TRUE—The scalene muscle, by elevating the 1st and 2nd ribs, sternum and clavicle, assists in forced inspiration. Reference *E*, p. 130.

144.3
TRUE—The external intercostal muscles, by elevating the ribs, assist in inspiration. Reference *E*, p. 130.

145.1
FALSE—The inferior vena cava and branches of the right phrenic nerve pass through the vena caval opening. Reference *E*, p. 129.

145.2
FALSE—The oesophagus passes through the oesophageal opening. Reference *E*, p. 129.

145.3
TRUE—The thoracic duct accompanies the aorta and the azygos vein through the aortic opening of the diaphragm. Reference *E*, p. 129.

146.1
FALSE—Spindle-shaped cells are a characteristic of smooth or involuntary muscle. Reference *K*, p. 26.

146.2
TRUE—Each muscle fibre of voluntary muscle is surrounded by a membrane called the sarcolemma. Reference *K*, p. 26.

146.3
TRUE—Each muscle fibre has several nuclei situated just under the sarcolemma. Reference *K*, p. 26.

2.5 ANGIOLOGY

147 Which of the following statements applies to the ophthalmic artery?

1. It enters the orbit through the optic canal (foramen).
2. It is a branch of the internal carotid artery.
3. It supplies the retina.

148 The arch of the aorta gives rise directly to the:

1. right common carotid artery.
2. right subclavian artery.
3. left subclavian artery.

149 Arteries arising from the external carotid artery include the:

1. superior thyroid artery.
2. lingual artery.
3. ophthalmic artery.

150 The immediate branches of the coeliac axis include the:

1. left gastric artery.
2. hepatic artery.
3. splenic artery.

Answers overleaf

147.1
TRUE—The ophthalmic artery enters the orbit through the optic canal. Reference *U*, p. 601.

147.2
TRUE—The ophthalmic artery is a branch of the internal carotid artery, given off just as the carotid leaves the cavernous sinus. Reference *U*, p. 601.

147.3
TRUE—The ophthalmic artery supplies the retina via its branch the central artery of the retina. Reference *U*, p. 601.

148.1
FALSE—The right common carotid artery is a branch of the brachiocephalic artery. Reference *D*, pp. 492 and 494 (Fig. 21–4).

148.2
FALSE—The right subclavian artery is the other branch of the brachiocephalic artery. Reference *D*, pp. 492 and 494 (Fig. 21–4).

148.3
TRUE—The left-subclavian artery is the third branch directly off the arch of the aorta. Reference *D*, pp. 492 and 494 (Fig. 21–4).

149.1
TRUE—The superior thyroid artery is an anterior branch of the external carotid artery, supplying the thyroid gland and larynx. Reference *U*, p. 603.

149.2
TRUE—The lingual artery is an anterior branch of the external carotid artery. Reference *U*, pp. 602 (Fig. 907) and 604.

149.3
FALSE—The ophthalmic artery is a branch of the internal carotid artery. Reference *U*, p. 601.

150.1
TRUE—The left gastric artery is an immediate branch of the coeliac axis. Reference *D*, p. 496.

150.2
TRUE—The common hepatic artery is one of the three immediate branches of the coeliac axis. Reference *D*, p. 496.

150.3
TRUE—The splenic artery is an immediate branch of the coeliac axis. Reference *D*, p. 496.

151 Arteries arising from the abdominal aorta include the:

1. lumbar.
2. coeliac.
3. superior mesenteric.

152 The veins of the arm include the:

1. brachial vein.
2. cephalic vein.
3. median cubital vein.

153 The great (long) saphenous vein:

1. lies anterior to the medial malleolus.
2. begins on the medial side of the ankle.
3. joins the popliteal vein.

Answers overleaf

151.1
TRUE—The left and right lumbar arteries are parietal branches of the abdominal aorta. Reference *D*, pp. 496 and 497 (Fig. 21–6).

151.2
TRUE—The coeliac artery is the first visceral branch of the abdominal aorta. Reference *D*, pp. 496 and 497 (Fig. 21–6).

151.3
TRUE—The superior mesenteric artery is a visceral branch of the abdominal aorta. Reference *D*, pp. 496 and 497 (Fig. 21–6).

152.1
TRUE—The brachial vein is a deep vein of the arm and accompanies the artery of the same name. Reference *D*, pp. 502 and 503 (Fig. 21–10).

152.2
TRUE—The cephalic vein is a superficial vein of the arm commencing from the dorsal arch of the hand and passing up the lateral border of the arm to join the axillary vein. Reference *D*, pp. 502 and 503 (Fig. 21–10).

152.3
TRUE—The median cubital vein connects the cephalic and basilic veins across the anterior surface of the elbow, and is a suitable vein for puncture. Reference *D*, pp. 502 and 503 (Fig. 21–10).

153.1
TRUE—The great saphenous vein lies anterior to the medial malleolus. Reference *D*, pp. 506 and 507 (Fig. 21–12).

153.2
TRUE—The great saphenous vein commences on the medial side of the ankle as a continuation of the medial end of the dorsal venous arch of the foot. Reference *D*, pp. 506 and 507 (Fig. 21–12).

153.3
FALSE—The great saphenous vein empties into the femoral vein in the groin. Reference *D*, pp. 506 and 507 (Fig. 21–12).

2.6 RETICULO-ENDOTHELIAL SYSTEM

154 Lymph from the right side of the head, neck and thorax drains into the:

1. thoracic duct.
2. cisterna chyli.
3. right lymphatic duct.

155 Lymph nodes contain:

1. phagocytic reticular cells.
2. lymphocytes.
3. macrophages.

156 The coeliac lymph nodes receive efferent vessels from the:

1. gastric lymph nodes.
2. pancreaticosplenic lymph nodes.
3. hepatic lymph nodes.

Answers overleaf

154.1
FALSE—The thoracic duct receives lymph from the left side of the head, neck and chest, the left upper extremity, and the entire body below the ribs. Reference *D*, pp. 527 and 528 (Fig. 22–5).

154.2
FALSE—Lymph from the left and right lumbar trunks and the intestinal trunk drains into the cisterna chyli. Reference *D*, pp. 527 and 528 (Fig. 22–5).

154.3
TRUE—The right lymphatic duct drains lymph from the upper right side of the body. Reference *D*, pp. 525 (Fig. 22–1(b)) and 528.

155.1
TRUE—Fixed phagocytic reticular cells line the sinuses of a lymph node. Reference *D*, p. 526.

155.2
TRUE—Lymph nodes contain lymphocytes in the lymph nodules. Reference *D*, pp. 525 and 526 (Fig. 22–3(a)).

155.3
TRUE—Macrophages are large phagocytic cells that can be found in lymph nodes. Reference *D*, p. 526.

156.1
TRUE—The gastric lymph nodes, draining the abdominal oesophagus, the stomach and the first part of the duodenum pass lymph to the coeliac lymph nodes. Reference *M*, p. 793.

156.2
TRUE—The pancreaticosplenic lymph nodes lie along the splenic arteries and the efferent vessels pass to the coeliac nodes. Reference *M*, p. 793.

156.3
TRUE—The hepatic lymph nodes, associated with the hepatic arteries pass lymph to the coeliac lymph nodes. Reference *M*, p. 793.

157 The functions of the spleen include:

1. destruction of red blood cells.
2. storage of red blood cells.
3. formation of antibodies.

158 Reticulo-endothelial cells are found in:

1. bone marrow.
2. the spleen.
3. the liver.

Answers overleaf

157.1
TRUE—The spleen is a site for the destruction of old red blood cells and removal of the breakdown products. Reference *D*, p. 538.

157.2
TRUE—The spleen stores and releases red blood cells in case of demand. Reference *D*, p. 538.

157.3
TRUE—The lymphoid tissue in the spleen is a site of antibody formation. Reference *D*, p. 545.

158.1
TRUE—Bone marrow contains reticulo-endothelial cells responsible for the formation of erythrocytes. Reference *F*, p. 9.

158.2
TRUE—The spleen contains reticulo-endothelial cells to produce antibodies and lymphocytes. Reference *F*, p. 157.

158.3
TRUE—The Kupffer cells, which partly line the liver sinusoids, are phagocytic reticulo-endothelial cells. Reference *F*, p. 154.

2.7 NEUROLOGY (GENERAL)

159 Cerebrospinal fluid is located in the:

1. subarachnoid space.
2. central canal of the spinal cord.
3. cerebral ventricles.

160 The brain and spinal cord are surrounded by the:

1. pia mater.
2. subarachnoid space.
3. dura mater.

161 The corpus callosum:

1. lies inferior to the falx cerebri.
2. is composed of white matter.
3. connects the two cerebral hemispheres.

Answers overleaf

159.1
TRUE—The subarachnoid space, between the arachnoid and pia mater, contains cerebrospinal fluid. Reference *O*, pp. 248 and 250.

159.2
TRUE—The central canal of the spinal cord contains cerebrospinal fluid. Reference *O*, p. 250.

159.3
TRUE—Cerebrospinal fluid is found in the cerebral ventricles. Reference *O*, p. 250.

160.1
TRUE—The pia mater is the innermost of the meninges that surrounds the brain and spinal cord. Reference *O*, pp. 248 and 249.

160.2
TRUE—The subarachnoid space, between the arachnoid and pia mater, surrounds the brain and spinal cord. Reference *O*, pp. 248 and 249.

160.3
TRUE—The dura mater, the outermost of the meninges, surrounds the brain and spinal cord. Reference *O*, pp. 248 and 249.

161.1
TRUE—The falx cerebri lies in the longitudinal fissure between the two cerebral hemispheres and inferior to it is the corpus callosum. Reference *D*, pp. 334 (Fig. 14–4) and 336.

161.2
TRUE—The corpus callosum is composed of white matter. Reference *D*, p. 336.

161.3
TRUE—The corpus callosum is a large bundle of transverse fibres connecting the two cerebral hemispheres. Reference *D*, pp. 334 (Fig. 14–4) and 336.

162 The spinal cord is transmitted through the:

1. vertebral foramen.
2. intervertebral foramen.
3. transverse foramen.

163 Structures which pass through the superior orbital fissure include the:

1. optic nerve.
2. trochlear nerve.
3. occulomotor nerve.

164 Sympathetic fibres of the autonomic nervous system:

1. cause dilation of the coronary arteries.
2. decrease the force of contraction of the heart.
3. increase secretions of the pancreas.

Answers overleaf

162.1
TRUE—The vertebral foramen of each vertebra contribute to the vertebral (spinal) canal to accommodate the spinal cord. Reference *D*, pp. 300 and 301 (Fig. 13–1).

162.2
FALSE—The intervertebral foramen formed between adjacent vertebrae permits the passage of the spinal nerves. Reference *D*, pp. 161 (Fig. 7–12(b)) and 162.

162.3
FALSE—The transverse foramen in each cervical transverse process is for the passage of the vertebral artery and vein. Reference *D*, p. 162 (Fig. 7–13).

163.1
FALSE—The 2nd cranial (optic) nerve passes through the optic foramen. Reference *O*, pp. 130 and 268.

163.2
TRUE—The 4th cranial (trochlear) nerve passes through the superior orbital fissure to supply the superior oblique muscle of the eye. Reference *O*, p. 130.

163.3
TRUE—The 3rd cranial (occulomotor) nerve passes through the superior orbital fissure to supply some of the external eye muscles. Reference *O*, pp. 130 and 268.

164.1
TRUE—One effect of the stimulation of the sympathetic fibres of the autonomic nervous system is to cause dilation of the coronary arteries. Reference *O*, p. 313.

164.2
FALSE—Decreased strength of the heartbeat is effected by the parasympathetic fibres. Reference *O*, p. 313.

164.3
FALSE—Parasympathetic fibres are responsible for effecting increased secretion of the pancreas. Reference *O*, p. 313.

165 Nerves supplying the tongue include the:

1. maxillary nerve.
2. facial nerve.
3. glossopharyngeal nerve.

166 The cerebellum is situated:

1. in the posterior cranial fossa.
2. below the cerebrum.
3. in front of the pons and medulla.

167 Which of the following functions are mainly attributed to the cerebellum?

1. Maintenance of balance.
2. Rate of respiration.
3. Vision.

Answers overleaf

165.1
FALSE—The maxillary nerve (part of trigeminal) supplies sensory fibres for the mucosa of the nose, palate, parts of the pharynx, upper teeth and lip, cheek and lower eyelid. Reference *D*, p. 347.

165.2
TRUE—The sensory fibres of the facial nerve are from the taste buds of the anterior two-thirds of the tongue. Reference *D*, p. 348.

165.3
TRUE—The sensory fibres of the glossopharyngeal nerve are from the taste buds on the posterior third of the tongue. Reference *D*, p. 348.

166.1
TRUE—The cerebellum, with the pons and medulla, is contained within the posterior cranial fossa. Reference *E*, p. 23.

166.2
TRUE—The cerebellum is located just below the posterior part of the cerebrum. Reference *O*, pp. 263 (Fig. 9–12) and 271.

166.3
FALSE—The cerebellum is posterior to the pons and medulla. Reference *O*, p. 263 (Fig. 9–12).

167.1
TRUE—The cerebellum controls skeletal muscles to maintain equilibrium. Reference *O*, p. 272.

167.2
FALSE—The rate of respiration is controlled by the medulla, peripheral chemoreceptors and the cerebral cortex. Reference *O*, pp. 544 and 545.

167.3
FALSE—Vision is the function of the visual cortex of the occipital lobes of the cerebrum. Reference *O*, pp. 336 and 337 (Fig. 11–21).

168 The 8th cranial nerve, vestibulocochlear (auditory) nerve:

1. is entirely a sensory nerve.
2. leaves the petrous portion of temporal bone through the internal acoustic (auditory) meatus.
3. is concerned with the appreciation of spatial position.

169 The medulla oblongata is continuous with the:

1. cerebrum.
2. pons.
3. spinal cord.

170 The spinal nerves include:

1. 8 pairs of cervical nerves.
2. 12 pairs of thoracic nerves.
3. 6 pairs of lumbar nerves.

Answers overleaf

168.1
TRUE—The two divisions of the 8th cranial nerve are both sensory. Reference *O*, p. 270.

168.2
TRUE—The internal acoustic (auditory) meatus, on the posterior portion of the petrous temporal bone, transmits the 8th cranial nerve. Reference *O*, p. 131 (Table 5–3).

168.3
TRUE—One of the functions of the 8th cranial nerve is the appreciation of the body in space as part of balance or equilibrium. Reference *O*, p. 266 (Table 9–4).

169.1
FALSE—The midbrain and the pons varoli are between the cerebrum and the medulla oblongata. Reference *K*, pp. 177 and 178.

169.2
TRUE—The pons is continuous with the midbrain above and the medulla oblongata below. Reference *K*, p. 178.

169.3
TRUE—The medulla oblongata extends from the pons above and is continuous with the spinal cord below. Reference *K*, p. 178.

170.1
TRUE—There are 8 pairs of cervical nerves. Reference *O*, pp. 256 and 259 (Table 9–3).

170.2
TRUE—There are 12 pairs of thoracic nerves. Reference *O*, pp. 256 and 259 (Table 9–3).

170.3
FALSE—There are only 5 pairs of lumbar nerves. Reference *O*, pp. 256 and 260 (Table 9–3).

171 The hypothalamus:

1. is a collection of grey matter.
2. forms the floor of the third ventricle.
3. activates the anterior lobe of the pituitary.

172 The cerebrospinal fluid:

1. is formed in the lateral ventricles.
2. passes into the subarachnoid space through holes in the roof of the fourth ventricle.
3. passes from the third ventricle to the fourth ventricle through the interventricular foramen.

Answers overleaf

171.1

TRUE—The hypothalamus consists of several structures composed of nerve cells (grey matter) situated beneath the thalamus and above the pituitary gland. Reference *O*, p. 273.

171.2

TRUE—The hypothalamus forms the floor of the third ventricle and the lower part of its side wall. Reference *O*, p. 273.

171.3

TRUE—Some of the axons of the hypothalamus secrete releasing hormones into the blood which control the release of certain anterior pituitary hormones. Reference *O*, p. 274.

172.1

TRUE—Cerebrospinal fluid is formed by the choroid plexuses in the lateral ventricles and also in the third and fourth ventricles. Reference *O*, p. 250.

172.2

TRUE—Cerebrospinal fluid passes through openings in the roof of the fourth ventricle, two laterally placed and one in the midline, into the cisterna magna, which is continuous with the subarachnoid space. Reference *O*, p. 250.

172.3

FALSE—The passage from the third ventricle into the fourth is called the cerebral aqueduct. The interventricular foramen is between each lateral ventricle and the third ventricle. Reference *O*, p. 250.

2.8 NEUROLOGY (SPECIAL SENSES)

173 The contents of the middle ear include the:

1. cochlea.
2. semicircular canals.
3. auditory ossicles.

174 The middle ear communicates with the inner ear via the:

1. fenestra vestibuli.
2. auditory (Eustachian) tube.
3. tympanic membrane.

175 The end organ of hearing:

1. is called the organ of Corti.
2. consists of hair cells.
3. is situated in the semicircular canals.

Answers overleaf

173.1

FALSE—The cochlea forms part of the bony labyrinth of the internal ear. Reference *O*, pp. 340 and 341 (Table 11–6).

173.2

FALSE—The semicircular canals form part of the structures of the internal ear. Reference *O*, pp. 340, 341 (Table 11–6) and 342.

173.3

TRUE—The middle ear, an air-filled cavity within the temporal bone, contains the three auditory ossicles. Reference *O*, pp. 338 (Fig. 11–22) and 339.

174.1

TRUE—The fenestra vestibuli (oval window) is a small opening between the middle and inner ear. The base of the stapes is held in it by ligaments and muscles. Reference *D*, pp. 401 and 403 (Fig. 17–11).

174.2

FALSE—The auditory tube connects the middle ear with the nose and nasopharynx. Reference *D*, p. 400 (Fig. 17–9(b)).

174.3

FALSE—The tympanic membrane lies between the external auditory meatus and the middle ear. Reference *D*, pp. 399 and 400 (Fig. 17–9).

175.1

TRUE—The organ of Corti is the organ of hearing in the cochlear duct. It consists of epithelial cells lying on the basilar membrane. Reference *D*, 402 (Fig. 17–10(d)).

175.2

TRUE—The organ of Corti consists of hair cells, the receptors of auditory sensations, and supporting cells. Reference *D*, p. 402 (Fig. 17–10(d)).

175.3

FALSE—The end organ of hearing is in the cochlear duct, part of the cochlea. Reference *D*, pp. 401 (Fig. 17–10(c)) and 402.

176 The olfactory nerve is:

1. a sensory nerve.
2. concerned with the sense of smell.
3. the 3rd cranial nerve.

Answers overleaf

176.1
TRUE—The olfactory (1st cranial) nerve is a sensory nerve. Reference *O*, pp. 266 (Table 9–4) and 268.

176.2
TRUE—The olfactory nerve is responsible for relaying the sensations relating to smell via the olfactory bulb and tract to the sensory areas located in the temporal lobe of the cerebrum. Reference *D*, pp. 341 and 346.

176.3
FALSE—The olfactory is the 1st cranial nerve, the occulomotor is the 3rd cranial nerve. Reference *O*, p. 268.

2.9 RESPIRATORY SYSTEM

177 The trachea can correctly be described as:

1. commencing at CV6
2. bifurcating at TV5.
3. lying behind the oesophagus.

178 During inspiration, the:

1. heart rate decreases.
2. diaphragm descends.
3. ribs move upwards and outwards.

179 The lungs are associated with which of the following functions of the body?

1. External respiration.
2. Fluid loss.
3. Temperature regulation.

Answers overleaf

177.1
TRUE—The trachea commences at the lower border of the cricoid cartilage at the level of CV6. Reference *J*, pp. 58 and 60 (Fig. 23).

177.2
TRUE—The trachea divides at the level of the sternal angle (TV5) into the right and left main bronchi. Reference *J*, pp. 58 and 60 (Fig. 23).

177.3
FALSE—The trachea lies in front of the oesophagus. Reference *D*, pp. 558 (Fig. 23–3) and 562.

178.1
FALSE—In most adults the heart rate does not alter during quiet breathing. In children, young adults and adults during deep voluntary breathing, the heart rate increases during inspiration and decreases during expiration. This is termed sinus arrhythmia. Reference *B*, p. 159.

178.2
TRUE—As the diaphragm contracts it descends, and increases the vertical diameter of the thorax. Reference *O*, p. 530.

178.3
TRUE—The ribs move upwards and outwards due to the contraction of the external intercostal muscles during inspiration. Reference *O*, p. 530.

179.1
TRUE—External respiration is the exchange of oxygen and carbon dioxide between alveolar air and pulmonary capillaries. Reference *D*, pp. 575 and 576.

179.2
TRUE—Fluid loss via the lungs is about 300 ml/day. Reference *D*, p. 696.

179.3
TRUE—Respiration assists in evaporation of water to remove heat from the body. Reference *D*, p. 660.

180 The vocal folds are attached to the:

1. cricoid cartilage.
2. thyroid cartilage.
3. arytenoid cartilages.

181 The trachea is:

1. continuous with the nasopharynx.
2. lined by squamous epithelium.
3. anterior to the oesophagus.

182 The rate of respiration is controlled by the:

1. carbon dioxide level in the blood.
2. medulla oblongata.
3. hypoglossal nerve.

Answers overleaf

180.1
FALSE—The vocal folds, two folds of mucous membrane with cord-like free edges, are not attached to the cricoid cartilages. Reference *K*, pp. 96 and 97 (Fig. 7:13).

180.2
TRUE—The vocal folds are attached to the inner wall of the laryngeal prominence of the thyroid cartilage anteriorly. Reference *K*, p. 97 (Fig. 7:13).

180.3
TRUE—The vocal folds are attached to the arytenoid cartilages posteriorly. Reference *K*, p. 97 (Fig. 7:13).

181.1
FALSE—The trachea is a continuation of the larynx. Reference *K*, pp. 94 (Fig. 7:7) and 97.

181.2
FALSE—The trachea is lined with pseudo-stratified ciliated columnar epithelium containing globlet cells. Reference *K*, p. 98.

181.3
TRUE—The trachea is anterior to the oesophagus. Reference *K*, p. 98.

182.1
TRUE—The partial pressure of carbon dioxide in the blood is one mechanism for controlling the respiration rate. Reference *K*, p. 105.

182.2
TRUE—The respiratory centre in the medulla oblongata is responsible for nervous control of inspiration. Reference *K*, pp. 104 and 105 (Fig. 7:25).

182.3
FALSE—The hypoglossal nerve is the motor nerve for the muscles of the tongue and hyoid bone. Reference *K*, pp. 192 and 193 (Table 12:3).

183 The thyroid cartilage:

1. lies opposite the second cervical vertebra.
2. forms the laryngeal prominence anteriorly.
3. has the vocal cords attached to its inner surface.

184 The cricoid cartilage has facets for articulation with the:

1. arytenoid cartilages.
2. thyroid cartilage.
3. epiglottis.

Answers overleaf

183.1
FALSE—The thyroid cartilage lies opposite the 4th and 5th cervical vertebrae. Reference *K*, pp. 94 (Fig. 7:7) and 95.

183.2
TRUE—The laryngeal prominence is the anterior part of the thyroid cartilage. Reference *K*, pp. 95 and 96 (Fig. 7:8).

183.3
TRUE—The vocal cords are attached to the inner surface of the thyroid cartilage anteriorly. Reference *K*, p. 97 (Fig. 7:13).

184.1
TRUE—The posterior part of the cricoid cartilage has articular areas for the arytenoid cartilages superiorly. Reference *K*, p. 96 (Fig. 7:9).

184.2
TRUE—The cricoid cartilage has articular areas for the thyroid cartilages inferiorly. Reference *K*, p. 96 (Fig. 7:9).

184.3
FALSE—The epiglottis is attached to the inner surface of the anterior wall of the thyroid cartilage immediately below the thyroid notch. Reference *K*, p. 96.

2.10 ALIMENTARY SYSTEM

185 The functions of the large intestine include:

1. secretion of bile.
2. desaturation of fats.
3. absorption of water, glucose and salts.

186 The common bile duct:

1. grooves the posterior surface of the head of pancreas.
2. passes behind the first part of the duodenum.
3. is formed by the union of the cystic and common hepatic ducts.

187 The lesser curvature of the stomach:

1. is a site for ulcers and cancers.
2. is connected to the lesser omentum.
3. has an angular notch two-thirds down its length.

Answers overleaf

185.1
FALSE—The liver is responsible for the secretion of bile. Reference *K*, p. 138.

185.2
FALSE—Desaturation of fats, conversion of stored fat into a form suitable for oxidation, is a function of the liver. Reference *K*, pp. 136 and 147.

185.3
TRUE—Absorption of water, glucose and mineral salts is a function of the large intestine. Reference *K*, p. 141.

186.1
TRUE—The common bile duct passes downwards in close proximity to the posterior surface of the head of pancreas. Reference *K*, pp. 136 and 137 (Fig. 9:36).

186.2
TRUE—The common bile duct passes behind the first part of the duodenum as it descends towards the duodenal papilla. Reference *K*, pp. 136 and 137 (Fig. 9:36).

186.3
TRUE—The cystic and common hepatic ducts unite to form the common bile duct. Reference *K*, p. 136.

187.1
TRUE—The lesser curvature of the stomach is the second most common site for peptic ulcers and gastric cancer, the most common site being the pyloric region. Reference *Q*, pp. 188 and 190.

187.2
TRUE—The peritoneal layers come together at the lesser curvature of the stomach and extend upwards to the liver as the lesser omentum. Reference *K*, p. 129 (Fig. 9:24A).

187.3
TRUE—The junction of the body and pyloric antrum of the stomach meet at the lesser curvature of the stomach and produce a notch. Reference *K*, p. 129.

188 Papillae located on the superior aspect of the tongue are:

1. vallate.
2. fungiform.
3. filiform.

189 Which of the following statements apply to the vermiform appendix?

1. It arises from the ileum.
2. It forms the ileocaecal valve.
3. It lies in the right iliac fossa.

190 The inner lining of the stomach wall:

1. is a thick layer of mucous membrane.
2. folds into rugae when the stomach is empty.
3. contains glands which secrete mucus, acid and pepsinogen.

Answers overleaf

188.1
TRUE—The vallate papillae form an inverted V-shaped row on the posterior part of the superior aspect of the tongue. Reference *O*, pp. 555 and 556 (Fig. 19–3A).

188.2
TRUE—Fungiform papillae are found on the sides and apex of the tongue. Reference *O*, pp. 556 (Fig. 19–3A) and 558.

188.3
TRUE—Filiform papillae are distributed over the anterior two-thirds of the tongue. Reference *O*, pp. 556 (Fig. 19–3A) and 558.

189.1
FALSE—The vermiform appendix arises from the caecum about 3 cm below the ileocaecal valve. Reference *O*, pp. 575 (Fig. 19–23) and 584.

189.2
FALSE—The ileocaecal valve is formed where the ileum joins the large intestine at the junction of the caecum and ascending colon. Reference *O*, pp. 574 and 575 (Fig. 19–23).

189.3
TRUE—The vermiform appendix lies in the right iliac fossa. Reference *O*, pp. 566 (Fig. 19–14) and 574.

190.1
TRUE—The inner lining of the stomach is a thick layer of mucous membrane. Reference *O*, p. 554 (Table 19–1).

190.2
TRUE—The inner lining forms rugae when the stomach is empty. These allow for distention. Reference *O*, pp. 554 (Table 19–1) and 568 (Fig. 19–16).

190.3
TRUE—The inner lining contains numerous coiled tubular gastric glands which secrete mucus, hydrochloric acid and pepsinogen. Reference *O*, pp. 569, 570 (Fig. 19–18) and 595 (Table 20–2).

191 Digestion is effected by enzymes which are secreted by the:

1. salivary glands.
2. gastric glands.
3. pancreatic glands.

192 The production of saliva is usually increased by which of the following stimuli?

1. Sight, smell and taste of food.
2. Atropine.
3. Fear.

193 The ileum:

1. is supplied by branches of the inferior mesenteric artery.
2. has a large aggregate of lymph follicles (Peyer's patches).
3. has a mesentery.

Answers overleaf

191.1
TRUE—The salivary glands secrete saliva which contains ptyalin, an amylase. Reference *O*, pp. 558 and 595 (Table 20–2).

191.2
TRUE—Gastric glands secrete pepsinogen, a precursor of the enzyme pepsin. Reference *O*, pp. 569 and 595 (Table 20–2).

191.3
TRUE—Pancreatic glands secrete proteases, lipase and amylase. Reference *O*, p. 595 (Table 20–2).

192.1
TRUE—The reflex mechanisms that control saliva secretion include the sight, smell and taste of food. Reference *O*, p. 598.

192.2
FALSE—Atropine blocks the visceral effectors of the autonomic nervous system and tends to decrease saliva production. Reference *O*, pp. 311 and 313 (Table 10–3).

192.3
FALSE—Fear results in increased epinephrine secretion by the adrenal medulla, which causes a decrease in saliva production. Reference *O*, pp. 313 (Table 10–3) and 379.

193.1
FALSE—The ileum, together with the duodenum, jejunum and the proximal half of the large intestine, is supplied by branches of the superior mesenteric artery. Reference *K*, pp. 76 and 77 (Fig. 5:37).

193.2
TRUE—The ileum has a large number of aggregated lymph follicles (Peyer's patches) towards the distal end. Reference *K*, p. 133.

193.3
TRUE—A double layer of peritoneum called the mesentery attaches the ileum and jejunum to the posterior abdominal wall. Reference *K*, p. 132.

194 When a patient is given a fatty mixture to drink, which of the following physiological functions occur?

1. The sphincter of Oddi opens.
2. The lining of the duodenum produces a hormone.
3. The gall bladder contracts.

195 Bile enters the duodenum through the:

1. duodenal papilla.
2. hepatopancreatic ampulla (of Vater).
3. pyloric sphincter.

196 Which of the following are within the substance of the parotid gland?

1. The maxillary artery.
2. The facial nerve.
3. The internal jugular vein.

Answers overleaf

194.1
TRUE—The sphincter of Oddi, a valve in the common bile duct, opens due to hormonal release from the intestinal mucosa when fat is present. Reference *D*, p. 627 (Exhibit 24–4).

194.2
TRUE—The intestinal mucosa produces a hormone, cholecystokininpancreozymin when fat is present in the duodenum. Reference *D*, p. 627 (Exhibit 24–4).

194.3
TRUE—The gall bladder contracts and ejects bile into the duodenum under hormonal control. Reference *D*, p. 627 (Exhibit 24–4).

195.1
TRUE—Bile enters the duodenum through an elevation of the duodenal mucosa known as the duodenal papilla. Reference *D*, pp. 615 and 616 (Fig. 24–12).

195.2
TRUE—The common bile duct unites with the pancreatic duct and enters the duodenum as the ampulla of Vater. Reference *D*, pp. 615 and 616 (Fig. 24–12).

195.3
FALSE—The pyloric sphincter guards the entrance of the pylorus of the stomach into the duodenum. Reference *D*, pp. 611 and 612 (Fig. 24–11(a)).

196.1
TRUE—The maxillary artery, a terminal branch of the external carotid artery is formed within the parotid gland and passes out of the gland on its anteromedial surface. Reference *M*, p. 1273.

196.2
TRUE—The facial nerve passes through the parotid gland as the main divisions of the buccal and mandibular branches. Reference *M*, p. 1273.

196.3
FALSE—The internal jugular vein runs downwards in the neck medial to the sternocleidomastoid muscle, a superficial muscle of the neck. Reference *K*, pp. 73 and 280 (Fig. 18:1).

197 The main functions of the liver include:

1. secretion of bile.
2. production of plasma proteins.
3. secretion of lipase.

Answers overleaf

197.1
TRUE—The liver cells synthesise the constituents of bile which pass into the bile ducts within the liver lobule. Reference *K*, pp. 135 (Fig. 9:34) and 136.

197.2
TRUE—The liver forms plasma proteins from amino acids. Reference *K*, p. 136.

197.3
FALSE—Lipase is produced in the pancreas and not in the liver. Reference *K*, pp. 137 and 138.

2.11 URINARY SYSTEM

198 The ureters:

1. are retroperitoneal structures.
2. enter the bladder anteriorly.
3. pass posteriorly to the iliac vessels.

199 The left ureter:

1. passes in front of the pancreas.
2. passes behind the second part of the duodenum.
3. has three coats only, mucous, muscular and fibrous.

200 Substances reabsorbed from the glomerular filtrate by the convoluted tubules include:

1. creatinine.
2. radiological contrast agents.
3. glucose.

Answers overleaf

198.1
TRUE—The ureters lie behind the parietal peritoneum on the posterior abdominal wall. Reference *O*, p. 660.

198.2
FALSE—The ureter openings lie at the posterior corners of the triangular-shaped floor (the trigone) of the bladder. Reference *O*, p. 661.

198.3
FALSE—The ureters pass anteriorly to the iliac vessels. Reference *O*, p. 639 (Fig. 22–1).

199.1
FALSE—Both the ureters and the pancreas are retroperitoneal structures, but the left ureter does not pass in front of the pancreas. Reference *O*, pp. 578 (Fig. 19–26) and 584.

199.2
FALSE—The second part of the duodenum descends on the right side of the median plane, the left ureter is 5 cm to the left at the same level. Reference *J*, pp. 74 (Fig. 35) and 81 (Fig. 43).

199.3
TRUE—The ureters have three coats: a lining of mucous membrane, a middle smooth muscle layer, and an outer fibrous coat. Reference *O*, p. 660.

200.1
FALSE—Creatinine is found in the glomerular filtrate, but is not reabsorbed by the convoluted tubules and appears as a constituent of urine. Reference *F*, pp 135 and 137.

200.2
FALSE—Radiological contrast agents that are capable of being excreted in the glomerular filtrate are not reabsorbed. Reference *V*, p. 291.

200.3
TRUE—Glucose is completely reabsorbed under normal conditions. Reference *F*, p. 137.

201 Functions of the kidney include:

1. storage of glycogen.
2. excretion of salts.
3. regulating the pH of the blood.

Answers overleaf

201.1
FALSE—Glycogen is stored in the liver and muscles. Reference *F*, p. 112.

201.2
TRUE—Inorganic salts, either as dissociated ions or soluble compounds, are excreted in the urine. Reference *F*, p. 139.

201.3
TRUE—The kidney is capable of excreting surplus hydrogen or hydroxyl ions as part of the pH regulation of blood. Reference *F*, pp. 138 and 140.

2.12 REPRODUCTIVE SYSTEM

202 The spermatic cord includes the:

1. testicular artery.
2. ductus (vas) deferens.
3. testicular vein.

203 Ovarian function is controlled by:

1. follicle stimulating hormone.
2. lactogenic hormone.
3. oxytocin.

Answers overleaf

202.1

TRUE—The testicular artery descends through the inguinal canal within the white fibrous cylindrical casing known as the spermatic cord. Reference *O*, p. 727 (Fig. 26–11).

202.2

TRUE—The ductus (vas) deferens ascends from the scrotum and passes through the inguinal canal as part of the spermatic cord. Reference *O*, pp. 724 and 727 (Fig. 26–11).

202.3

TRUE—The testicular vein, represented by the pampiniform plexus, ascends the inguinal canal as part of the spermatic cord. Reference *O*, p. 727 (Fig. 26–11).

203.1

TRUE—Follicle stimulating hormone stimulates several primary ovarian follicles into growth at the commencement of the ovarian cycle. Reference *D*, pp. 727 (Fig. 28–17) and 728.

203.2

FALSE—Lactogenic hormone initiates milk secretion after the mammary glands have been prepared by a number of other hormones. Reference *D*, p. 416.

203.3

FALSE—Oxytocin stimulates uterine contraction and the contractile cells around the ducts of the mammary glands. Reference *D*, p. 418.

2.13 ENDOCRINE SYSTEM

204 Endocrine cells within glands:

1. empty their secretions along short ducts.
2. produce enzymes.
3. produce hormones.

205 The islets of Langerhans:

1. are located in the pancreas.
2. produce insulin.
3. pass their secretions down the pancreatic duct.

206 Which of the following exhibit an endocrine function?

1. Pancreas.
2. Testes.
3. Placenta.

Answers overleaf

204.1
FALSE—Endocrine glands have no ducts but secrete their products into the interstitial fluid or blood. Reference *O*, p. 62.

204.2
FALSE—Enzymes, organic catalysts, influence chemical reactions either intracellularly or, in the case of digestive enzymes, extracellularly. Reference *O*, p. 594.

204.3
TRUE—Endocrine glands produce hormones which influence various structures and functions. Reference *O*, pp. 349 and 350.

205.1
TRUE—The islets of Langerhans are within the substance of the pancreas. Reference *O*, pp. 379, 380 and 584.

205.2
TRUE—Insulin is produced by the beta cells within the islets of Langerhans. Reference *O*, pp. 380 and 584.

205.3
FALSE—The secretions from the islets pass into the blood capillaries within the pancreas and not via the duct system of the pancreas. Reference *O*, pp. 388 and 584.

206.1
TRUE—The pancreas exhibits an endocrine function via the islets of Langerhans. Reference *O*, p. 584.

206.2
TRUE—The testes perform an endocrine function through the secretion of the male hormone, testosterone. Reference *O*, p. 720.

206.3
TRUE—The placenta performs a temporary endocrine function during pregnancy, producing chorionic gonadotropins, oestrogen and progesterone. Reference *O*, p. 382.

207 The medulla of the suprarenal gland produces:

1. adrenalin.
2. hydrocortisone.
3. adrenocorticotrophic hormone (ACTH)

208 Features of thyrotoxicosis are:

1. an excess of thyroxine.
2. a deficiency of aldosterone.
3. a slow pulse rate.

209 Secretions of the anterior lobe of the pituitary gland include:

1. follicle stimulating hormone (FSH).
2. growth hormone (GH).
3. antidiuretic hormone (ADH).

Answers overleaf

207.1
TRUE—Adrenalin (epinephrine) is produced by the medulla of the suprarenal gland upon sympathetic neurone stimulation. Reference *K*, p. 223.

207.2
FALSE—Hydrocortisone (cortisol) is a glucocorticoid secreted by the suprarenal cortex. Reference *K*, p. 222.

207.3
FALSE—Adrenocorticotrophic hormone (ACTH) is secreted by the anterior lobe (adenohypophysis) of the pituitary gland. Reference *K*, pp. 218 and 219.

208.1
TRUE—Abnormally high amounts of thyroxine lead to a disorder referred to as thyrotoxicosis. Reference *I*, pp. 217 and 218.

208.2
FALSE—A deficiency of aldosterone (produced by the adrenal cortex) would lead to Addison's disease. Reference *I*, p. 222.

208.3
FALSE—A feature of thyrotoxicosis is a rapid pulse rate. Reference *I*, p. 218.

209.1
TRUE—Follicle stimulating hormone (FSH) is one of the gonadotrophic hormones secreted by the anterior lobe of the pituitary gland. Reference *K*, pp. 218 and 219.

209.2
TRUE—Growth hormone (GH) is secreted by the anterior lobe of the pituitary gland. Reference *K*, p. 218.

209.3
FALSE—Antidiuretic hormone (ADH) or vasopressin is a secretion of the posterior lobe (neurohypophysis) of the pituitary gland. Reference *K*, p. 220.

2.14 SURFACE MARKINGS AND LEVELS, REGIONS AND RELATIONS

210 A transverse section of the abdomen between the 1st and 2nd lumbar vertebrae would show the:

1. duodenum.
2. stomach.
3. left kidney.

211 Structures seen on a transverse section through the body at the level of the 10th thoracic vertebra include the:

1. right kidney.
2. oesophagus.
3. spleen.

212 Which of the following structures are found in the hypogastrium?

1. The fundus of the stomach.
2. The urinary bladder.
3. The rectum.

Answers overleaf

210.1
TRUE—The duodenum is at the level of L1–L2 (transpyloric plane). Reference *J*, pp. 68 (Fig. 30) and 74 (Fig. 35).

210.2
TRUE—The stomach lies at the level between L1 and L2 (transpyloric plane). Reference *J*, pp. 68 (Fig. 30) and 73 (Fig. 34).

210.3
TRUE—The left kidney would be visible on a transverse section between the 1st and 2nd lumbar vertebrae. Reference *J*, p. 80 (Fig. 42).

211.1
FALSE—The upper limit of the right kidney is at a level of T11–12 disc space. Reference *J*, p. 80 (Fig. 42).

211.2
TRUE—The oesophagus is passing through the oesophageal opening of the diaphragm at this level. Reference *J*, pp. 59 (Fig. 22) and 72.

211.3
TRUE—The spleen can be sectioned at the level of T10 and would lie to the left side and posteriorly. Reference *W*, p. 74 (Fig. 11.1).

212.1
FALSE—The fundus of the stomach lies in the left hypochondrial region of the abdomen. Reference *J*, pp. 68 (Fig. 30) and 72.

212.2
TRUE—The urinary bladder is situated in the hypogastrium and the fundus extends upwards in the umbilical region when distended. Reference *J*, pp. 68 (Fig. 30) and 81.

212.3
TRUE—The rectum is situated in the hypogastrium. Reference *J*, p. 80 (Fig. 41).

213 Structures located behind the peritoneum include the:

1. abdominal aorta.
2. pancreas.
3. suprarenal glands.

214 The position of the thymus gland in the thoracic cavity is:

1. posterior to the trachea.
2. partly in the superior mediastinum
3. more anterior than the arch of the aorta.

215 Structures anterior to the right kidney include the:

1. spleen.
2. duodenum.
3. hepatic flexure of the colon.

Answers overleaf

213.1
TRUE—The abdominal aorta and all its main branches are retroperitoneal. Reference *P*, pp. 128 (Fig. 83) and 180.

213.2
TRUE—The pancreas is located behind the peritoneum. Reference *P*, pp. 121 and 180.

213.3
TRUE—The suprarenal glands, situated above the upper poles of the kidneys, are located behind the peritoneum. Reference *P*, pp. 125, 126 (Fig. 81) and 180.

214.1
FALSE—The thymus gland is anterior to the trachea, being directly posterior to the sternum. Reference *D*, pp. 429 (Fig. 18–20) and 538.

214.2
TRUE—The thymus gland lies partly in the superior mediastinum and partly in the anterior mediastinum. Reference *D*, pp. 15 (Fig. 1–4) and 429 (Fig. 18–20).

214.3
TRUE—The thymus gland is more anterior than the arch of the aorta. Reference *P*, p. 24 (Fig. 17).

215.1
FALSE—The spleen is posterolateral to the left kidney. Reference *D*, pp. 538 and 622 (Fig. 24–15).

215.2
TRUE—The second part of the duodenum is anterior to the right kidney. Reference *D*, p. 622 (Fig. 24–15).

215.3
TRUE—The hepatic flexure of the colon is anterior to the right kidney. Reference *P*, p. 126 (Fig. 81).

REFERENCES

A Gibson J. (1981). *Modern Physiology and Anatomy for Nurses*, 2nd edn. Oxford: Blackwell Scientific Publications.

B Macdonald Critchley. ed. (1978). *Butterworths Medical Dictionary*, 2nd edn. London: Butterworths.

C Govan A.D.T., MacFarlane P.S., Callander R. (1981). *Pathology Illustrated*. Edinburgh: Churchill Livingstone.

D Tortora G.J., Anagnostakos N.P. (1981).*Principles of Anatomy & Physiology*, 3rd edn. New York: Harper and Row.

E Bryan G.J. (1982). *Radiographic Skeletal Anatomy*, 2nd edn. Edinburgh: Churchill Livingstone.

F Green J.H. (1983). *An Introduction to Human Physiology*, 4th edn. Oxford: Oxford University Press.

G Gunn C. (1984). *Bones and Joints*. Edinburgh: Churchill Livingstone.

H Romanes G.J. (1979). *Cunningham's Manual of Practical Anatomy*, 14th edn., volume 3. Oxford: Oxford University Press.

I Davies P.M. (1985). *Medical Terminology*, 4th edn. London: William Heinemann Medical Books.

J McKears D.W., Owen R.H. (1979). *Surface Anatomy for Radiographers*. Bristol: John Wright and Sons.

K Wilson K.J.W. (1981). *Foundations of Anatomy and Physiology*, 5th edn. Edinburgh: Churchill Livingstone.

L Romanes G.J. (1978). *Cunningham's Manual of Practical Anatomy*, volume 2, 14th edn. Oxford: Oxford University Press.

M Williams P.L., Warwick R. (1980). *Gray's Anatomy*, 36th edn. Edinburgh: Churchill Livingstone.

N Schlossberg L., Zuidema G.D. (1980). *John Hopkins Atlas of Human Functional Anatomy*. Baltimore: John Hopkins University Press.

O Anthony C.P., Thibodeau G.A. (1983). *Textbook of Anatomy and Physiology*, 11th edn. St Louis: CV Mosby Co.

P Ellis H. (1983). *Clinical Anatomy*, 7th edn. London: Blackwell Scientific Publications.

Q Thomson A.D., Cotton R.E. (1983). *Lecture Notes on Pathology*, 3rd edn. London: Blackwell Scientific Publications.

References

R Passmore R., Robson J.S. Editors-in-Chief. (1976). *A Companion to Medical Studies*, volume 1, 2nd edn. London: Blackwell Scientific Publications.

S McKears D.W., Owen R.H. (1979). *Surface Anatomy for Radiographers*. Bristol: John Wright and Sons.

T Hamilton W.J., Simon G., Hamilton S.G.I. (1971). *Surface and Radiological Anatomy*, 5th edn. Cambridge: W. Heffer and Sons Ltd.

U Lockhart R.D., Hamilton G.F., Fyfe F.W. (1965). *Anatomy of the Human Body*, 2nd edn. London: Faber and Faber Ltd.

V Bryan G.J. (1979). *Diagnostic Radiography*, 3rd edn. Edinburgh: Churchill Livingstone.

W Kreel L. ed. (1979). *Medical Imaging*. Aylesbury: HM and M Publishers Ltd.

Titles of related interest: